THE ILLNESS IS THE CURE

THE ILLNESS IS THE CURE

Second extended edition

an introduction to
LIFE MEDICINE &
LIFE DOCTORING

a new existential approach to illness

Peter Wilberg

© Peter Wilberg 2012, 2nd extended edition 2014.

Published by New Yoga Publications, Whitstable, Great Britain

ISBN-13: 978-1500263720
ISBN-10: 1500263729

Disclaimer

This radical critique of biological medicine is in no way intended to invalidate the good intent and caring efforts of countless physicians, nurses and other health professionals operating within institutions dominated by the biomedical belief system.

Its only aim is to help release them – and their patients – from the iron grip of that system. Nor does this book seek to deny the role either of emergency care or surgery, or natural forms of symptomatic relief known and used for centuries (in particular remedies such as aspirin whose source lies in natural plant extracts).

Finally, this book is certainly not a critique of patients who continue to have trust in biomedical tests and treatments – and/or suffer little side effects from them. For though such treatments, for example pharmaceutical treatments and radiotherapy, may carry very serious dangers, they can also serve as a form of psychological as well as biological medicine.

Contents

Introduction

Questions for the Reader

Have you ever felt that by simply making an appointment to see your doctor you are just bothering them and interfering with their busy schedule?

Have you ever felt your doctor's sole purpose in listening to you is to come to the quickest possible way of seeing you out – whether by handing out a prescription or arranging a test?

Have you ever felt frustrated by the lack of truly patient listening time that doctors are able or willing to give you?

Have you ever felt infantilised or treated like a child by medical professionals?

Have you ever felt that there was no time for your questions to be fully heard or answered?

Have you ever felt confused by often dramatically conflicting opinions and beliefs expressed by different doctors and consultants?

Have you ever felt frustrated about being given one medical test after another, being passed from one anonymous consultant to another, or being given one form of treatment or surgery after another – all without ever having a say in what is going on?

Have you ever felt that your direct felt experience of your illness was of no interest to medical professionals or 'experts'?

Have you ever felt so scared by a medical diagnosis such as cancer that it has made you feel ill – even though you might have been feeling fine or even had absolutely no symptoms at all beforehand?

Have you ever suffered acute or chronic side effects from medical drugs and treatments that you were not warned about – or that were largely ignored?

Have you ever wondered at the high cost of health insurance, drugs and treatments – and why it is that even publicly funded health institutions and services are constantly in financial crisis?

Has it ever occurred to you that illness is a source of huge profits for drug companies, the corporate health industry as a whole, and even promoters of health 'supplements' or 'alternative' medicine?

Have you ever considered that illness itself may at least partly be an expression of life as people are economically pressured to live it in a fundamentally sick and money-driven society?

Have you ever suspected that the timing and nature of your illness was not accidental but had to do with events that had been going on in your life and feelings associated with them?

Have you ever felt, as a medical practitioner, that there may be a lot more to a patient's symptoms or illness than meets the medical eye – but that your training has not equipped you to explore it, and that your job and institutional environment give you no time or encouragement to do so?

If so, then read on....

Guiding Thoughts

"Disease occurs ... not in the body but in life."

J. Good Byron,

"The idea of one basis for Science and another for Life is from the very outset a lie." *Karl Marx*

"It is far more important that one's life should be perceived than it be transformed; for no sooner has it been perceived than it transforms itself of its own accord."

Maurice Maeterlinck

"An advanced industrial society is sick-making because it disables people from coping with their environment and, when they break down, it substitutes a 'clinical' prosthesis for the broken relationships."

"People would rebel against such an environment if medicine did not explain their biological disorientation as a defect in their health, rather than as a defect in the way of life which is imposed on them or which they impose on themselves."

"A number of authors have ... tried to debunk the status of mental deviance as a 'disease'. Paradoxically, they have rendered it more and not less difficult to raise the same kind of question about disease in general."

Ivan Illich

"Patients turn their problems into illnesses, and ... the physician's job is to turn them back into problems."

Michael Balint

"...the body's symptoms are not necessarily pathological, that is, they are not just sicknesses which must be healed, repressed or cured. Symptoms are potentially meaningful and purposeful conditions... as well as a royal road into the development of the personality."

Arnold Mindell

"A psychological medicine ... obviously comes into conflict with the technological development of medicine, which has already become an Über-technology. This development is itself closely connected with modern economic structures, with industry, with the income sources of physicians, with the gigantic need for patients – and others – to be deceived."

"That illnesses have meaning, can lead those affected to the meaning of their lives – this is the insight that natural-scientific medicine has fundamentally impeded."

"One sees, now, that psychology in medicine brings forth an unexpected result. It does not only bring knowledge of the soul, but illuminates the body in such a way as to let it appear in a new light. The body is no longer what it seemed before, and what anatomy and physiology teach."

"Illness can be experienced as this – that through a bodily occurrence a development in awareness is created."

"The greatest goal would be to understand how in every case, in what way an illness is just a muted final thought, a still insufficiently [fulfilled] creative act."

Viktor von Weizsäcker

"... health is not an objective condition which can be understood by the methods of natural science alone. It is rather a condition related to the mental attitude by which the individual has to value what is essential for his life. 'Health' ... consists in the individual's capacity to actualise his nature to the degree that, for him at least, is essential." *Kurt Goldstein*

"... scientific determinism is the root and prevalent philosophy in our present Western technological culture, where the bulk of our endeavours incline to engineering, that is, the direct alteration and control of physical structures. Medical practice, deriving from this outlook, is based on the assumption that distress can only be alleviated by changing behavioural or physical manifestations of that distress. Antacids for dyspepsia, tranquillizers for anxiety, and behaviour therapy for sexual dysfunction are clinical examples of this engineering philosophy. The experience of distress, it is held, will yield to control of its physical determinants; there is no need to explore or amplify the experience itself, as the experience is only a reflection of disturbed underlying mechanism."

David Zigmond

"... science is, to a quite unimaginable degree, through and through dogmatic; dealing with un-thought-through conceptions and preconceptions. It is of the highest importance that there be thinking physicians, who are not of a mind to leave the field for the scientific technologists."

"... the genetic approach is clear to everyone. It seems self-evident. But it suffers from a deficit, which is all too easily and therefore all too often overlooked. To be in a position to explain an illness genetically, we need first of all to explain what the illness in itself is."

"Those who wish to stick rigidly to genetic explanation, without first of all clarifying the essence of that which they wish to explain, can be compared to people who wish to reach a goal, without first of all bringing this goal in view."

"All explanation reaches only so far as the explication of that which is to be explained."

"It can be that a true understanding of the essence of an illness...prohibits all causal-genetic explanation...."

Martin Heidegger

"If people become ill, it is quite fashionable to say that the immunity system has temporarily failed – yet the body itself knows that certain 'dis-eases' are healthy reactions. The body does not recognise diseases as diseases in usually understood terms."

"You are not healthy … no matter how robust your physical condition, if your relationships are unhealthy, unsatisfying, frustrating or hard to achieve."

"…a person in poor health <u>should be</u> seen by the physician in relationship to the family and also in relationship to the environment. Old-time family doctors understood the patient's sensitivity to family members and to the environment, of course, and they often felt a lively sympathy and understanding that the practitioners of modern medicine often seem to have forgotten."

"…try to understand that the particular dilemma of illness is not an event forced upon you … Rather realise that to some extent or another your dilemma or your illness <u>has been chosen by you</u>…

"There is no need to feel guilty since you <u>meant very well</u> as you made each choice…"

"… no person dies ahead of his or her time. The individual chooses the time of death."

"…no individual dies of cancer or AIDS, or any other condition, until they themselves have set the time."

from *The Way Toward Health – a Seth book by Jane Roberts*

"Through the long succession of millennia, man has not known himself physiologically; he does not know himself even today."

Friedrich Nietzsche

"The 'I' is first and foremost a bodily 'I'."

Sigmund Freud

The Basic Questions

- What if 'explaining' an illness is one thing, but *understanding* it is quite another?
- What if illnesses have *life meanings* and not just biological 'explanations' and 'causes'?
- What if the *biology* of the human body cannot be separated from the *biography* of the human being?
- What if *the life of the human body* cannot in any way be separated from *the life of the human being* in all its existential dimensions – personal, social and economic?
- What if *body symptoms* are like *dream symbols* – there to be understood and to tell us something?
- **What if 'the illness is the cure'** – offering patients an opportunity to gain important insights into themselves to bring about healing transformations in their *lives* and not just their bodies?
- What if conventional biomedical tests and treatments aimed at finding ways to fight and 'cure' a person's illness can prevent them from learning vital lessons from their illness?
- What if official medical statistics show that conventional forms of biomedical treatment are themselves a leading cause of death ?
- What if many prescription drugs worsen or prolong the very symptoms they are prescribed for?
- What if so-called 'scientific' medicine is really *money-driven medicine* – relying on illness as a cash cow for the corporate health industry?
- What if every *bodily state* is at the same time a *state of consciousness* – and vice versa – thus making nonsense of the separation between 'body' and 'mind', medical treatments on the one hand and psychological therapies on the other?

Then we would need a new understanding of illness and a new model of medicine – one that not only questions but goes beyond the biomedical model.

- This in turn could spare both individuals and private and public health services the huge costs of pharmaceutical drugs and hi-tech biomedical equipment.
- It would also mean that psychological counsellors and therapists could no longer leave 'medical' problems and symptoms to the medical profession.
- Indeed it would allow a new foundation for *medical training* to be created – not biological medicine but 'Life Medicine'.
- Out of this could come very different ways of treating patients – not through conventional doctoring but through 'Life Doctoring'. For the aim of Life Medicine and the Life Doctor is to help patients discover in what ways their *illness is the cure* – there to help them *heal their lives.*
- In this way the individual patient would no longer be reduced to 'a case' of some generic 'disease'. Instead every such 'case' and every such 'disease' would be understood in terms of the individual life circumstances behind it.

Medicine, Life and Science

In a way intended to be of help to both patients and health professionals, this book challenges one of the most basic assumptions shared by almost *all* forms of medicine – conventional or 'alternative', 'scientific', 'traditional' or 'spiritual'. This is the assumption that illness is something to *be cured* rather than *being the cure*.

To challenge this basic assumption, I introduce a fundamentally new 'existential' approach to health and illness which I call 'Life Medicine' and 'Life Doctoring'. Life Doctoring and Life Medicine offer patients opportunities to come to an understanding of how and in what ways their *illness is itself the cure* – offering a source of new *healing understandings* of themselves and a *healing transformation* of their lives.

For in contrast to both 'orthodox' and 'alternative' medicine – each of which in their own ways seek nothing but 'causes' and 'cures' for illness – Life Medicine and Life Doctoring do not *separate* science and life, biology from biography, the life of the *human body* and the life of the *human being*. Instead the focus is on the larger *life context* and *specific life meanings* that particular symptoms and illnesses hold for the individual patient. For as Marx wrote:

"The idea of one basis for science and another for life is from the very outset a lie."

This 'lie' unfortunately has dire consequences of which too few are aware. For research by the medical establishment itself has shown that conventional biomedical diagnosis and treatment through drugs and surgery is itself *the* leading cause of premature death – ahead of both cancer and heart disease.

By offering an entirely new framework for understanding health and illness, Life Medicine and Life Doctoring can help patients to not only understand the underlying sense of 'dis-ease' in their *lives* that lies behind their illness. Life Medicine and Life Doctoring can also serve a vital *preventative* role by (a) preventing this 'dis-ease' manifesting further as clinical 'disease', and (b) educating patients about the possible dangers and potentially sickness-causing or 'iatrogenic' effects of many standard forms of biomedical testing and treatment.

Both biomedical and 'alternative' explanations of illness are comparable in many respects to the way in which scientists sought to 'explain' dreams before Freud – denying them all *meaning*. Yet what if the symptoms are comparable to disturbing dream symbols and experiences – both expressions of a felt 'dis-ease '? What if illnesses are a type of embodied dream or 'body dream'? Then deep *understanding* and not just medical-scientific 'explanation', testing and treatment is required.

For again, to 'explain' an illness is one thing. Yet to *understand* it is quite another. For understanding has to do with *meaning*. Yet so-called 'biological' medicine does not even recognise or understand the root meaning of the very term 'biology' itself – which does not refer to a set of specialist sciences, but rather to the 'speech' (Greek *logos*) of 'life' (Greek *bios*). Speech carries and communicates meaning. Nothing could be further from the root meaning of 'biology' then, than the so-called biological 'sciences' – which reduce the life, language and 'speech' of the human body itself to a mere molecular 'expression' of its genes.

That is why, as Martin Heidegger wrote: *"The essential realm in which biology moves can never be grounded in biology as a science."* For the realm in which biology moves is a realm of living and embodied meaning. In contrast, what most fundamentally defines the 'biomedical model' of medicine – based as it is on "biology as a science" – is the way it totally denies any *personal life meaning* to illness – and in particular the exact timing, life situation and larger life context in which an individual's symptoms first emerge. On the contrary, by merely seeking to fit a person's symptoms into the frame of wholly impersonal diagnostic or statistical criteria, and then treating their illness with no less impersonal methods of drug or hi-tech treatment, biomedicine can *aggravate* the very sense of *personal meaning loss* that lies behind most illnesses – as well as damaging rather than healing patients' bodies, and even endangering their lives.

The continuing *monopoly* of biomedicine over our entire understanding of and approach to illness has one reason and one reason only – namely that it is not actually 'science driven' but 'money driven' – turning illness into a source of vast profits for the drug companies and manufacturers of hi-tech medical equipment. Indeed 'health' itself is increasingly defined merely in monetary terms – as the patient's capacity for 'employment' as a wage-slave and to 'function' economically as a profit-source for employers.

Many people are concerned about the rising costs of public health care or angered by a global trend towards the privatisation of health services. Yet the roots of this trend lie in the fact that *illness itself* has long been 'privatised' – seen as bearing no relation at all to the social and economic 'ills' affecting the patient. To declare that 'the illness is the cure' is also to recognise that the 'cause' of illness does not lie in the individual alone but also in the world – and that illness itself is in part a *healthy* response to a fundamentally *sick world* – and this way also helps to *heal* that world.

On Biological Medicine

Medicine and Meaning

"Modern medical science largely considers the human body to be a kind of mechanical model, a sort of vehicle like a car that needs to be checked by a garage every so often."

from *The Way Toward Health* by Jane Roberts

A driver who for some reason is in a hurry to get somewhere decides to 'run the red light' at a junction, and has an accident. Yet would we even think of seeking to explain their consequent injuries purely as a result of automobile mechanics, for example suspecting the possibility of 'faulty pedals' or some other mechanical defect – seeing this as what 'caused' the car to go through the red light (and then subjecting the car to a whole series of diagnostic tests).* This would seem absurd to common sense – and yet it is no less absurd than seeing the body as a mechanical vehicle – like a car – and treating illness as something caused by a technical fault in some part of that vehicle.

For cars also have drivers. To be sure, the driver in our example made a choice, whereas we do not normally think of ourselves as 'choosing' to get ill. Yet the driver's choice itself was no doubt a response to a current or overall *life situation*. The driver might have been in a hurry for some reason, for example late for work or for a job interview. The decision to run the red light may not even have been a fully conscious or premeditated decision – simply a more or less aware bodily reaction to the specific life situation itself. Nevertheless shooting the red light was a choice.

What if the same applies to illness? Namely that there is a way in which we do not so much consciously 'choose' as subconsciously 'accede' to getting ill, albeit in a particular life context and for particular life reasons that are quite conscious to us: for example a pressing need to get a job – or even a subconscious desire to use the illness as a way of taking 'time out' from the pressures of life and/or receiving care and attention. Whatever the possible *meaning* of the accident/illness might be for a specific individual there is one thing we can be sure of however – there *is* such a meaning – and that just seeking, however thoroughly, for a mechanical fault in the individual's bodily 'vehicle' *will never reveal it.*

Indeed even *were* such a mechanical fault to be discovered or diagnosed, it might itself be the result of a subconscious decision on the part of our 'driver' in response to a situation arising in their life journey i.e. something that in some way *drove* them to neglect that vehicle or ignore its warning signs. Simply taking the vehicle to a garage and repairing the fault will therefore not address its true meaning or that of its possible consequences. For these have to do with the life circumstances of the human being and not the mechanics or 'biology' of his bodily vehicle alone. Simply to say, for example, that the driver got a dodgy vehicle with an inherited 'fault', that they neglected it or abused it through mishandling – or that they failed to put it through a regular medical 'MOT' – is not enough. For the question 'why?' still remains – a question of life motive and meaning and not a mere matter of some inherited biological or mechanical 'defect', 'accident', or sequence of 'cause and effect'.

Even for our hypothetical driver who ends up in hospital due to a serious 'accident' the result might be a highly meaningful and life-changing one in a positive sense, allowing him or her to *re-think their life* and not just receive treatment for their body. Yet this simple but basic distinction – between the life of the human being and its expression in the life of the human body – is consistently ignored by medical science and biological medicine – which by seeking explanations for illness purely in terms of defects of our bodily 'vehicle' blocks all forms of research into the *meaning* of illness. For even if a defect is found in the form of some medically recognised 'disease' or 'disorder', biological medicine cannot yet explain the cause of the disease or disorder itself – except in terms of some genetic defect. Yet not even any form of genetic explanation can actually explain why one *individual and not another* should contract a particular disease. For just as not everyone who smokes gets lung cancer, and not everyone falls ill from an epidemic, neither does everyone with an errant gene end up with the disease associated with it.

*acknowledgement to Andrew Gara for this significant analogy

What Biological Medicine Can't Explain

The more biological medicine seeks to 'scientifically' explain illness – the more it leaves *unexplained.*

Examples:

Why medical treatment itself is a leading cause of death – ahead of cancer and heart disease.

Why most pharmaceutical drugs do not work on most of the patients they are designed for.

Why there is hardly a single class of pharmaceutical medication that doesn't have as a possible or even common 'side effect' a short- or long-term worsening of the symptoms it was prescribed for.

Why the majority of patients seen by doctors are made up by what they call 'the worried well' – in reality ordinary people who really wish to share psychological problems – life problems – with a professional, but wouldn't think of going to see a psychologist.

Why 'successful' drug treatment or surgery illness often precipitates mental psychosis or precedes the emergence of new symptoms just as serious as the original ones.

Why the greatest danger period for the mental and physical health patients occurs after finishing a' successful' course of medical treatment and being told that they are well.

Why social isolation is a greater risk factor for health and lowers life expectancy more than smoking, diet or obesity.

Why support groups for women with breast cancer patients have been found to double their life expectancy.

Why support from a spouse dramatically improves survival rates from heart transplants.

Why so many illnesses occur after or often on the exact anniversary of significant life events – such as bereavements, the end of a relationship, the start or loss of a job, taking an exam, retirement or even just going on holiday.

Why there is an 80% correlation between stressful life events and the onset of an illness in the two years following those events.

Why the chances of simply getting a cold are increased by life difficulties or disappointments, in particular those to do with employment or relationship problems.

Why the incidence of previously widespread, common and dangerous diseases was decline long before the use of antibiotics to treat them or the use of mass vaccinations to prevent them.

Why a study has shown that only 3.5% of the decline in mortality from infectious diseases can be attributed to drug treatments.

Why chemotherapy for all types of cancer is still used even though it has been shown by countless reports and admitted by many cancer specialists to be ineffective even in increasing life expectancy, and why death rates from cancer have actually increased with the increased use of chemotherapy.

Why, despite the Nobel Prize winning 'discovery' that the 'cause' of stomach ulcers was not 'stress' but a specific bacterium it was then found that between one and two-third of the world population carry this bacterium in their stomachs without developing ulcers.

Why 20-40% of children and 10% of adults carry the tuberculosis bacillus without contracting tuberculosis, and why only a minority of those exposed to the bacillus will develop TB.

Why children allergic to household dust at home showed no allergic responses when this dust was distributed in the hospital rooms.

Why Whitehall civil servants who are given orders by their superiors have twice the chance of contracting diabetes than those who give them their orders.

Why counselling for cardiac patients can prevent recurrence of heart attacks or even reverse arterial blockages, and why half of all heart attacks occur in people with normal cholesterol levels.

Why patients whose surgeons talk to them whilst under anaesthesia are at less risk of dying, and why patients whose surgeons openly discuss post-operative pain before surgery experience it less.

Why someone with sensitive skin can work for years with materials they are sensitive too, and yet only develop allergic reactions when emotional problems in their relational life flare up.

Why soldiers whose armies suffered defeat in battle were more likely to develop dysentery or typhus.

Why autopsies of thousands of young and otherwise healthy soldiers revealed atherosclerotic plaques of the sort generally associated only with older people, long-term smokers and others thought to be at risk of heart attacks and strokes from developing these plaques over time.

Why 'placebos' or fake surgery can be just as effective as 'active' drugs and real surgery.

Why people smoke, take illegal drugs, over- or under-eat, eat foods 'bad' for their health.

Why off-the-counter medications and legally prescribed drugs are a cause of greater and more widespread addiction – and often more difficult to come off – than illegal drugs.

Why people become obsessed with changing to or pursuing supposedly healthy 'lifestyles' through diets or fitness regimes – yet without ever really examining their lives as such and the health of their relationships.

Why both medical journals and the press are full of reports of new medical research and newly discovered dangers or aids to health – without ever asking what it means to be 'healthy'.

Why doctors will always ask patients 'how long' they have had a particular symptom but almost never ask WHEN it started, let alone what was going in the patient's life at the time – or in the days, weeks, months or years before the symptoms or symptoms appeared.

Why patients given home treatment after a heart attack have a lower mortality rate than those given impersonal, hi-tech hospital care.

Why patients with severe dementia, inability to speak and move – or despite almost complete destruction of their brains through cancer – have often been observed to sit up, move their limbs and speak with total clarity and rationally in the hours preceding their death.

Acknowledgements:

Why People Get Ill? by Darian Leader and Michael Cornfield, Hamish Hamilton 2007, for several of the examples included.

Getting Ill to See a Doctor

"The doctor is the drug."

"...the drug 'doctor' is a potent one with many unwanted side effects."

Michael Balint

In a society in which biological medicine or 'biomedicine' is institutionally dominant and 'mental illness' is still tainted by stigma, getting ill and seeing a doctor remains the principle *socially acceptable way* for people who are consciously or unconsciously ill-at-ease with their lives to obtain the care and attention they need or seek.

Precisely for this reason however, a *primary purpose* of illness can be to serve as a *principal communicative medium* by which individuals seek – through the clinical encounter with a physician – acknowledgement of their *existential* dis-ease or *life* suffering – one whose origin or 'etiology' does not lie in the biological life of the patient's body but rather in their *life as such* and their *life-world as a whole* (including their work world, family world etc).

However the *pre-condition* demanded by the clinical encounter for attaining the acknowledgement, care and attention that the patient seeks for their existential dis-ease is that they 'present' the physician with bodily symptoms that can be neatly fitted in the diagnostic schema of biomedicine, i.e., acknowledged as signs of recognised *diseases* for which standard biomedical tests and treatments can be prescribed. If this pre-condition is *not* fulfilled the individual risks being classed as a hypochondriac, malingerer or 'heart-sink' patient, i.e., one whose symptoms, old or new, consistently defy any form of straightforward clinical diagnosis, despite repeated visits to their doctor, multiple medical tests or appointments with specialist consultants.

For the individual *not* merely to be written off or classed as a hypochondriac or malingerer, *their own body knows full well* that it must translate or 'body forth' their existential dis-ease and life suffering in the form of symptoms of an 'actual' biological illness or disease capable of diagnostic identification and treatment.

The word 'iatrogenic' comes from the Greek words *genesis* (origin) and *iatros* (physician) and is used to refer to illnesses originating from medical treatment itself. One of the intrinsically *iatrogenic* dimensions of biological medicine lies in the fact that in many cases *patients do not simply go to doctors because they are ill.* Instead *they become ill in order to be able to go to doctors* – to create opportunities through the clinical encounter for the indirect communication and acknowledgment of their existential dis-ease and life suffering. This is perhaps the chief purpose and meaning of illness in the context of the clinical encounter.

Particularly in the case of individuals who are lonely or isolated, or whose communicative world or abilities do not fulfil their need to be understood, the clinical encounter with a physician is sought as something *intrinsically healing* – healing simply because of the opportunity it offers for a *tiny dose of understanding communication* – however medically distorted this 'understanding' may be and however absurdly time-limited the communication itself (in contrast, for example, to a 50 minute psychotherapy session).

It is the *modicum* of human contact provided by the clinical encounter with the physician or the human care provided by hospitalisation that is most healing for the patient. In this context, it would be most interesting to have available statistics showing the number of patients whose symptoms diminish or even disappear on the *very day* of an appointment with a doctor – feeling better simply through the expectation or experience of being able to *communicate* their suffering with a human being who is, by profession, duty bound to give them care and attention, take their suffering seriously and 'understand' it – even if only in biomedical terms.

Ivan Illich identified three types of iatrogenesis – clinical, social and cultural.

'Iatrogenesis is clinical when pain, sickness and death result from medical care ; it is social when health policies reinforce an industrial organization that generates ill-health; it is cultural and symbolic when medically sponsored behaviour and delusions restrict the vital autonomy of people by undermining their competence in growing up, caring for each other, and aging, or when medical intervention cripples personal responses to pain, disability, impairment, anguish and death.'

To the three types of iatrogenesis identified and described by Illich one could add a fourth. I call this 'communicative iatrogenesis'.

Communicative iatrogenesis arises from the fact that the required *language* necessary to seek and attain understanding communication through doctoring is the language of bodily *illness itself.* For whilst it would not be usual for a recently bereaved and lonely widow(er) to see a doctor in order to complain of being 'heart-broken' or of 'losing heart' to live, what *is* culturally acceptable – if not normative – is to go to a doctor and complain of pains in the region of the heart or heart arrhythmias. This is something that the patient knows. Yet – and this is the key factor – it is also something that the patient's *body* knows and is capable of responding to – by generating chest pains or heart arrhythmias. Of course there is such a thing now as 'bereavement counselling '. Yet how many prospective patients are informed or would be inclined to take it up – rather than seeing the very need for such counselling as a sign of emotional weakness.

36

Communicative iatrogenesis can be understood as a fundamental dimension of what Illich himself calls 'cultural and symbolic' iatrogenesis – biomedically diagnosable illness being a culturally determined and also symbolic *password* for obtaining the sought-after acknowledgement and communication of an individual's life suffering *through* that illness and in the *context* of the clinical encounter.

From this perspective, the 'ordinary' patient is just as much an individual in need of and in search of attention, care and communicative understanding as the 'heart-sink patient' or 'hypochondriac '. The distinction lies in the fact that the latter may ultimately fail to fulfil their needs through the clinical encounter. This is because they lack the central 'key' to obtaining the critical 'password' to it. This key is their willingness to *let* their own body translate or 'body forth' their existential disease or life suffering – not just in the form of medical *symptoms* but in the form of a 'genuine' – medically diagnosable – biological illness or disease.

In considering the origin or 'etiology' of illness from an existential and 'hermeneutic' perspective therefore – one that focuses on the *meaning* and *purpose* of illness rather than its biological 'causes' – we cannot exclude *the existential meaning of the clinical encounter for the patient* and the *purpose that illness serves within its* biomedical framework, i.e., as a necessary 'password' to that encounter and the opportunity it offers for fulfilling basic communicative needs.

The idea that becoming ill has a *meaning and purpose* is heretical enough in a cultural climate dominated by biological medicine. The sad paradox is that in such a culture the relational healing that patients seek through fulfilment of their basic human needs – for human contact, care and understanding communication – can be met only by getting *physically ill*. Thus whilst children are often understood to complain of symptoms or even to somehow 'actually' get ill as a way of seeking attention, the culture of biomedicine demands that *adults* do the same thing – simply in order to *call attention* to their existential dis-ease, their life suffering, stress or distress.

The Medical Consultation as a 'Set Up'

A patient wishes to *make sense* of his or her symptoms and arranges to see a doctor. So an appointment is duly made. Yet what remains unspoken in the consultation is that it is tacitly expected to take as its starting point certain unquestioned assumptions which serve as expected 'points of departure' for all doctor-patient communication. Below I list some of the most basic tacit assumptions that 'enframe' the medical consultation and constitute expected points of departure for all communication that occurs within it.

1. It is tacitly understood that we all know what 'illness' and 'health' are, that they are opposites, and that 'illness' is something 'bad' and 'health' something 'good'.

2. It is tacitly understood and agreed that the patient arranges the consultation because he is suffering symptoms of a possible 'illness' which he wishes to have identified and which he or she is therefore prepared to have diagnosed through examination and testing and be prescribed treatment for.

3. It is tacitly understood and agreed that the patient will describe their symptoms and that the physician will, directly or through further tests, arrive at a medical diagnosis of the disease, recommend a course of biomedical treatment aimed at relieving their symptoms or 'curing' the disease – based on knowledge of its biological 'causes'.

4. It is tacitly understood and agreed that the patient has just happened to fall victim to their symptoms 'out of the blue' – in other words that there is no meaning to be attached to the specific timing of their appearance in the larger context of the patient's life and life history.

5. It is tacitly understood and agreed therefore, that symptoms have no meaning at all beyond being mere signs of a possible biological disease or dysfunction.

6. It is tacitly understood and agreed therefore that 'making sense' of symptoms means nothing more than taking them as

possible signs of some biomedical disease – and that in no case can a biological illness or disease be itself taken as a symptom of a life-disease – a hidden life problem that manifests in the patient feeling 'ill-at-ease' with their lives.

7. It is tacitly understood and agreed that the patient's suffering – their felt pain, discomfort or 'dis-ease' – is a mere secondary and subjective 'effect' of an organic disorder or 'disease'. The contrary notion, namely that symptoms, illness and disease may be a symbol ic embodiment of a subjectively felt dis-ease' – and of particular ways in which the patient is 'ill-at-ease' with their life – is ruled out in advance. Indeed such a notion constitutes sheer heresy in terms of the unquestioned dogmas of biomedical 'science'.

Should a patient reject any or all of these assumptions, or depart from any of the unspoken rules or points of departure in their communication with a doctor, the patient will be immediately classed as a 'difficult' or 'incompliant' patient or even as deluded. Yet together these tacitly agreed assumptions and points of departure for a biomedical consultation effectively constitute an unspoken 'set up' or 'frame up' – a framework the patient is expected to compliantly adhere to. The aim of this 'frame up' is to enframe the meaning of the patient's symptoms in the terms of one framework only – that of biomedicine – excluding any other possible ways of making sense of those symptoms. Any attempt by a patient to question this framework – even if only by not immediately accepting certain types of routine biomedical tests or courses of treatment – will arouse indignation and bewilderment, be seen as a threat to the authority of biomedically trained doctors and a waste of the limited time they give to their patients. Instead it could be seen as an opportunity to give themselves more time to learn about the lives of their patients as human beings, to understand their symptoms in the larger context of their life and life world.

What Most Doctors Don't Ask

What follows is a list of some of the questions that most doctors don't ask – and yet which are key questions for both doctor and patient in coming to understand the life meaning of particular symptoms or a particular illness. They are the sort of questions central to Life Medicine and those that a Life Doctor will ask and discuss with you.

When did your symptoms first occur?

Is there anything else in your life that is bothering/distressing you right now?

What was going on in your life in the hours, days, weeks, months or years preceding the onset of your symptoms?

What were the most significant life encounters, events, experiences, dilemmas and decisions that faced you in the period preceding the onset of your symptoms?

What was the underlying mood you experienced in this period and how would you describe it?

What were the most dominant thoughts and emotions you experienced in this period?

What do you tend to think about most when you are most aware of your symptoms?

What feelings accompany these thoughts?

What do you do with those thoughts and feelings when you have them?

What do you tend to do in response to your symptoms themselves?

At what specific times or in what specific life situations do your symptoms tend to occur or intensify?

At what times or in what situations do your symptoms tend to disappear or diminish?

Have you experienced similar symptoms in the past, and if so at what times and in what circumstances?

How do your symptoms – and the thoughts you have around them – affect your emotional life, work and relationships?

What do your symptoms either force you to do or stop you from doing?

Is there any positive benefit you can see from the way your symptoms affect your life?

How would you describe the overall or underlying mood or state of consciousness accompanying your symptoms and/or the thoughts and emotions around them?

How do your symptoms make you feel? In what way does the mood that accompanies them affect not only what you think and how you feel but also who you are – your sense of 'you'?

Is there any positive side to the different mood and sense of self accompanying your symptoms?

Are there any other ways you could give expression to it in your way of relating to life and other people?

Alternatively, what changes in your way of relating to life and other people do you feel would most help to alter this underlying mood and/or alleviate your symptoms?

What are the most important types of experience you miss or have missed in your life and relationships?

What are the most important potentials or abilities you feel are not or have not been fulfilled or realised in your life?

What are the biggest fears or concerns you have about your symptoms, your illness or its treatment?

What would make you most happy or content in your life – independently of any improvement in your condition?

Empathy – a Foreign Language for Doctors?

(see also appendix 5)

It seems that most doctors literally cannot bring themselves to utter even the most *basic and commonplace empathic phrases* in response to a patient's presentation of his or her symptoms – even though these can have an immediately beneficial and healing impact. Indeed they are even taught in their medical training empathy as such is a hindrance to maintaining clinical 'objectivity' in doctor-patient communication. In reality it can be the magic key to affirming – rather than defending themselves against – the patient's lived, subjective *experience* of illness. In this way it can give an immediate sense of being recognised as a human being and with it an immediately enhance sense of well-being. In contrast, maintaining a stance of 'clinical distance' is a form of communicative pathology in the most literal sense– a 'sick' (*pathos*) use of language (*logos*). Yet since empathy is clearly a 'foreign language' for most biomedical doctors and clinicians what follows can be likened to a elementary language phrasebook, not in 'English as a Foreign Language' (EFL) but in 'Empathy as a Foreign Language' (EFL) one *so basic it is quite extraordinary that it should be needed at all.* Note: feel free to distribute or put a copy of it up for doctors in your local clinical practice or hospital!

1. Opening empathic phrases in response to patient's presentation:

For example, how about simple phrases like:

I'm sorry to hear that. / I'm sorry to hear you've been feeling that way/so bad.

That sounds very unpleasant/distressing/painful.

How has that been making you feel?

I can understand why you feel so worried/upset/concerned/distressed.

I can understand why you wanted to see me.

How have you been coping?

2. Some simple closing phrases to end a consultation:

How are you feeling now?

How do you think you will cope?

Do you have any other worries?

Is there anything else that you'd like to tell me about/ that is bothering you?

Do let me know how things go. (which the patient could do by leaving a note for their doctor by phone)

The common failure to use this type of empathic language is itself *symptomatic* of a larger problem – namely the almost total lack of interest on the part of clinicians in the patient's *lived experience* of illness and its effects *on* their life rather than *just* their presenting symptoms.

"One unintended outcome of the modern transformation of the medical care system is that it does just about everything to drive the practitioner's attention away from the experience of illness. The system thereby contributes importantly to the alienation of the chronically ill from their professional care-givers and, paradoxically, to the relinquishment by the practitioner of that aspect of the healer's art that is most ancient, most powerful and most existentially rewarding."

Arthur Kleinman M.D. *The Illness Narrative: suffering, healing and the human condition*

Automated Diagnosis and
the Future of Biomedicine

Have you ever wondered what is going on in your doctor's mind during a consultation? A large part of it is likely to be a process of observation, data gathering and analysis based – more or less accurately – on what you say. I emphasise the 'more or less' because many patients are surprised to see how often what they say to doctors is ignored or just plain misrepresented in their medical reports. And if, as Einstein noted in relation to physics, "Theory determines what is observed", then in the case of the 'observations' and 'data' gathered by the doctor in listening to you the same applies. Indeed it is often the case, paraphrasing Einstein, that in the case of biomedical practice 'Theory' determines not just what is 'observed' but even what is *heard* by doctors. The biomedical practitioner's chief aim is, like a radio, to distinguish 'signals' from 'noise' – 'noise' being anything the doctor regards as scientifically irrelevant to exercising his diagnostic skills – such as the larger life story behind a patient's illness, their emotional experience of illness – and of its effect on their life.

Yet what if what doctors are *chiefly* doing while listening to you is merely functioning as a human 'black box' between what *they* regard as significant 'input' and giving what they regard as all-important 'output', i.e. probable diagnoses, suggested treatments, prescriptions, referrals for further tests or to specialists? As this 'black box', what is really going on in your doctor's mind is comparable to them going through a type of predetermined computer 'algorithm' or 'decision tree' in order to arrive at the most likely or statistically probable 'diagnoses' from the 'observations' and 'data' he or she is collecting from you. In which case, however, the doctor is effectively functioning as nothing more than a sort of *human computer* – and therefore could just as well be ultimately replaced *by* a computer – one fitted out with what is called 'automated diagnostic software'. If you think this is a wild, futuristic idea – then think again. For 'Computer-Assisted Diagnosis' is already a reality – and is even used to get a 'second opinion' by the most highly revered of biomedical diagnosticians.

"At last he spoke. "Lymphoma with secondary hemophagocytic syndrome," he said. The crowd erupted in applause. Professionals in every field revere their superstars, and in medicine the best diagnosticians are held in particularly high esteem. Dr. Gurpreet Dhaliwal, 39, a self-effacing associate professor of clinical medicine at the University of California, San Francisco, is considered one of the most skilful clinical diagnosticians in practice today... Since medical school, he has been an insatiable reader of case reports in medical journals, and case conferences from other hospitals. To observe him at work is like watching Steven Spielberg tackle a script or Rory McIlroy a golf course. He was given new information bit by bit – lab, imaging and biopsy results. Over the course of the session, he drew on an encyclopedic familiarity with thousands of syndromes. He deftly dismissed red herrings while picking up on clues that others might ignore, gradually homing in on the accurate diagnosis."

Nevertheless the same New York Times report asked: "Just how special is Dr Dhaliwal's talent? More to the point, what can he do that a computer cannot?". It also acknowledged that even the famous Dr Dhaliwal "...occasionally uses a diagnostic checklist program called Isabel, just to make certain he hasn't forgotten something." It adds that the program has yet to offer a diagnosis that Dr Dhaliwal missed" – without saying whether this program could actually have done the same job as Dr Dhaliwal, and that in even less than the 45-

minutes he is given at medical conferences to display his showman-like skills in diagnosing "vexingly difficult cases".

Yet aside from a small number of diagnostic 'geniuses' and 'gurus' of the sort represented by Dr Dhaliwal (as well as in the fictional American TV series 'Dr House' – a doctor with similarly encyclopaedic knowledge of biomedicine and insatiable interest in the latest medical research), today there is not a doctor in the world, whether generalist or specialist, with a mental 'storage' space of enough encyclopaedic capacity or 'Gigabyte' equivalents to remember even what he or she learnt in their medical training – let alone find the motivation or time to keep up with the latest biomedical research. So we end up with a system whereby, reaching the limits of *his or her* knowledge, your doctor will refer you to a specialist of one sort or another – even though the knowledge of specialists too, is not encyclopaedic – and is no less innately limited by the interest in and time they have in keeping up with the latest research and developments in their field. Hence also the often diametrically opposed opinions that find expression among researchers and/or clinical practitioners *in the same specialty* – one hardly compatible with the smug complacency of doctors or specialists each of whom generally claim their own personal viewpoints, diagnoses or clinical judgements to be the most accurate or 'objective'.

The sad fact that comes to light here is that it is precisely *because* medical practice and the functioning of the medical mind takes data accumulated in the form of impersonal biomedical 'science', 'research ', 'evidence' and 'observations' as its diagnostic foundation, there is nothing that sophisticated diagnostic software with ever-larger databases of biomedical knowledge could not in fact *do better* than any human doctor – generalist or specialist. Given also that biomedicine effectively treats the human body as no more than a biological machine, much like a car, that may be in need of repair, it comes as no surprise to read the following arguments for a new 'Automated Medical Diagnosis System' – the aim of which is to eliminate "human bias" of any sort – even in using current forms of 'Computer Assisted Diagnosis':

"Cars can be plugged in at the mechanics for electronic diagnosis, customer issues logged in enterprise support systems receive immediate potential solutions to their issue prior to a customer service representative looking at it, and computers send error reports when an application crashes. In industries across the world automated diagnostics becomes more and more prevalent leveraging continually advancing algorithms that become increasingly intelligent in identifying solutions to known problems. Yet in the health care industry Doctors have outdated and limited access to potential solutions... *Enter symptom, disease type, test name or code* requests one physician diagnosis database. As with any human search that begins with keywords chosen by the user, bias inherently influences the results. If a Doctor has an assumed diagnosis, they will immediately begin searching for further evidence that their assumption can be validated. And if it isn't, then they will have missed other potential diagnoses. Additionally, if the Doctor begins searching by symptoms, while these may be accurate, the order or weight given to any one symptom will give a bias toward related diagnosis when in fact, there may be a symptom not given any credit and thus not included in the search. Regardless of whether you consider today's databases or the older process of researching in books, the results are always influenced by the bias of the researchers' initial assumptions. What is needed instead is an approach that minimizes human bias and considers all relevant and irrelevant data in determining a diagnosis. Computer software does this well."

"With an automated medical diagnosis system, Doctors could be presented with multiple potential diagnoses based on all of the patient's current and past details. Such a system could be designed for automated medical diagnosis that is based on probability, utility and decision theory."

"Essentially, the computer software could be fed human observations of symptoms, test results, and any machine data collected such as blood pressure, heart rate, oxygen levels, etc. The software would then compare these observations with a database of potential diseases and external agents (e.g. viruses, bacteria) to determine the most probable diagnosis. These results would then be presented back to the doctor along with a probability rating indicating which ones are likely most relevant or accurate. Each diagnosis could also then be presented with additional direction to the doctor to further explore for additional symptoms and/or order an additional test. These additional observations and/or test results would again then be fed into the system where it could re-evaluate the probable diagnoses cancelling out some while raising the probability of others. In addition to immediate interactions with the software, Intensive Care Unit's machine observation data (e.g., oxygen levels, heart monitors) could be constantly fed into the system to allow the software to be looking for patterns that match other known diagnosis that would never be able to be caught by a human as it would take too much time to evaluate the data."

What we are presented with here is indeed a futuristic image – albeit a dystopic one. Already hospitals and large clinical surgeries with multiple doctors have become, as Dr David Zigmond notes, more like airports than the so-called 'old-fashioned' surgeries run by family doctors – who knew their patients and their lives intimately. In contrast, in our clinical 'airports' you check in, go through a gate to see to see a doctor and check out with a prescription or referral for a further test of some sort or a consultation with a specialist.

For decades now, employment in manufacturing industries such as car-making has fallen through the introduction of robots that are pre-programmed to do the job required of them more precisely than any human worker could. Now however, we are confronted with the prospect of human beings, all seen as anonymous body-machines to be processed in automated high-tech hospital 'repair stations', and, as in some futuristic science fiction movie – conveyed on a factory-like medical conveyor belt. Stop one on the belt: patients' bodies are CCTV'd and perhaps even scanned in different ways while what they look like and say is digitally recorded to be searched for diagnostic signs, keywords and patterns. Stop 2: they are sent on a second conveyor line where blood tests or further scans are conducted automatically. Stop 3: they are either discharged from this fully automated hi-tech hospital 'garage' – where they are given any necessary drugs, a dose of radiotherapy, are either then conveyed to a stationary 'cubicle' for further processing – or else to an operating theatre 'manned' entirely by robots. And all this with the whole technological process merely supervised by a handful of technicians and actual human doctors. Finally, Stop 4: either a crematorium or a bill to be paid – as in coming to the exit barrier of a car park.

Not only is this science fantasy prospect a conceivable one – it is also an entirely *rational* one in the framework of biomedicine. Which only goes to show how totally *irrational* medical 'rationality' can be. For what this picture essentially lacks is what is most essential, not just to healing (as opposed to mere 'medicine ') but to human health *as such* – namely the care and care-giving of other *human beings* – not to mention truly *human* insight, observation, empathy, as well as human life experience and life understanding. On the other hand, it is *no less conceivable* that the development and refinement of 'automated medical diagnosis' could serve precisely to *free* doctors of the future from their current role as human computers, allowing them instead to devote most of their time and awareness to their human role as healer, care-giver or 'life doctor' – there to explore the patient's experience of illness and its *meaning* in the context of their lives and relationships – something no computer software or database will ever be able to do. In this way biomedical knowledge would find its true place as a tool subordinate to the *art* of healing – rather than becoming a substitute for that art. And since the terminology of biomedical science itself is as rich in metaphor as in 'fact', more precise and accurate biomedical diagnoses would also allow for more accurate and penetrating analyses of their own *symbolic* dimensions of meaning.

Until we reach this point however, next time you see a doctor bear in mind the question posed at the start – what is actually going on in the doctor's mind and what is he or she actually *there* for? For it will make a world of difference to your health whether the doctor is only there for a specific 'what' (for example, to go through a quasi-automated mental-diagnostic process and then refer you on for further medical processing) or whether the doctor is there for a very specific human being or 'who' – *for you.*

Reference:
Zigmond, David *If you want good personal Healthcare see a Vet*

How Biomedical Diagnosis
can Damage Your Health

Diagnostic screening

"Diagnosis may exclude a human being with 'bad' genes from being born, another from promotion, and a third from political life. The mass hunt for health risks begins with dragnets designed to apprehend those needing special protection ... Health testing ... was welcomed as the poor man's escalator into the world of Mayo [the Mayo Clinic] and Massachusetts General ... [yet] studies indicate that these diagnostic procedures – even when followed up by high-level medical treatments – have no positive impact on life-expectancy ... in any case, it transforms people who feel healthy into patients anxious for their verdict." *Ivan Illich*

Example: screening of men for higher than normal age-levels of PSA (Prostate Specific Antigen) of a sort which may indicate the presence of cancer of the prostate.

Diagnostic statistics

"By equating statistical man with biologically unique men, an insatiable demand for finite [medical] resources is created ... the right of the patient to withhold consent to his own treatment vanishes as the doctor argues that he must submit to diagnosis, since society cannot afford the burden of curative procedures that would be even more expensive."

Example: enormous pressure is placed on men with high PSA levels to undergo intrusive needle biopsies in order to extract cell samples for analysis and confirm the presence of cancerous cells – even though such biopsies produce many 'false negative' results, and even positive results allow no firm *prognostic* conclusions to be drawn whatsoever.

That is why one reading of the acronym PSA is 'Producer of Stress and Anxiety'.

Diagnostic screening statistics

Example: Two large, long-awaited studies [reported by the New England Journal of Medicine] failed to produce convincing evidence that routine prostate -cancer screening significantly reduces the chances of dying from the disease without putting men at risk for potentially dangerous and unnecessary treatment. The PSA blood test, which millions of men undergo each year, did not cut the death toll from the disease in the first decade of a U.S. government-funded study involving more than 76,000 men, researchers reported yesterday.

In the U.S. study, researchers randomly assigned 76,693 men ages 55 to 74 at 10 centres to receive either six annual screenings consisting of PSA testing and physical examinations or whatever their doctors recommend, which could include screening.

After seven years, 22 percent more prostate cancer s were diagnosed in the PSA group, and 17 percent more were diagnosed after 10 years. But there was no significant difference in deaths from the cancer in the two groups. The researchers noted there were actually more deaths overall in the screened group – 312 vs. 225 – and they could not rule out that the excess may have been the result of overtreatment.

The second study, a European trial involving more than 162,000 men that was released simultaneously, did find fewer deaths among those tested. But the reduction was relatively modest, and the study showed that the screening resulted in a large number of men undergoing needless, often harmful treatment. Stein, Rob *Philadelphia Inquirer*, 2009

Diagnostic stress and isolation

"Diagnosis always intensifies stress, defines incapacity, imposes inactivity, and focuses apprehension on non-recovery, on uncertainty and on one's dependence on future medical findings, all of which amounts to a loss of autonomy ... It also isolates a person in a special role, separates him from the normal and healthy, and requires submission to the authority of specialised personnel. Once a society organises for a preventative disease-hunt, it gives epidemic proportions to diagnosis. This ultimate triumph of therapeutic culture turns the independence of the average healthy person into an intolerable form of deviance." *Ivan Illich*

Example: the diagnosis of prostate cancer – like any form of cancer – produces an unhealthy degree of anxiety and stress, fear and uncertainty of a sort which makes the individual more likely to passively submit to medical authority and with it to dangerous and damaging forms of further diagnostic testing and/or treatments such as chemo- or radio-therapy – all of which, in the case of prostate cancer, drastically reduce quality of life whilst bringing no definitive 'cure' and often requiring further repeated and debilitating treatments.

Diagnostic error

"Diagnostic bias in favour of sickness combines with frequent diagnostic error. Medicine not only imputes questionable categories with inquisitorial enthusiasm; it does so at a rate of miscarriage that no court system could tolerate. In one instance, autopsies showed that more than half the patients who died in a British university clinic with a diagnosis of specific heart failure had in fact died of something else." (Illich, ibid.)

Example: many men die *with* prostate cancer even though they have not died from it.

Diagnostic damage and 'iatrogenesis'

Example: many forms of diagnostic testing are potentially dangerous and damaging in themselves. In the case of prostate cancer biopsies they not only accentuate the very symptoms that first led them to be done (e.g. urinary difficulties, production of blood in the urine) or produce infections of the prostate. Should cancerous cells be found, the biopsy procedure itself increases the likelihood of these cells spreading to other parts of the body – thus helping to realise the worst possible outcome and prognosis of a malignant tumour through the very procedure of diagnosis itself. In this way diagnosis itself becomes a form of *iatrogenesis* – medically generated disease. As for actual treatments of prostate cancer, in a large proportion of cases these can result not only in the generally debilitating effects of such therapies but also in permanent impotence.

When 'The Cure Becomes the Illness'

"The medical establishment has become a major threat to health. The disabling impact of professional control over medicine has reached the proportions of an epidemic. Iatrogenesis, the name for this new epidemic, comes from *iatros*, the Greek word for 'physician', and *genesis*, meaning 'origin'."

Ivan Illich *Medical Nemesis, The Expropriation of Health*

'Iatrogenesis' then, means 'originating from a physician' and refers to "preventable harm resulting from medical treatment or advice to patients. Professionals who may sometimes cause harm to patients are: physicians; pharmacists; nurses; dentists, psychologists, and therapists. Iatrogenesis can also result from complementary and alternative medicine treatments." (Wiki)

Medically caused or 'iatrogenic illness' is the elephant in the room as regards the whole domain of biomedicine. Hence the deafening silence when a study published in the Journal of the American Medical Association[1] reported that in the United States an estimated 225,000 deaths per year have iatrogenic causes, with only heart disease and cancer causing more deaths"[1] – making biomedicine itself the third leading cause of illness-related death. Since the publication of this studiously ignored article, new figures show that biomedicine may have become the leading cause of death (see appendix 3 on 'Death by Doctoring').

"Doctor-inflicted pain and infirmity have always been a part of medical practice. Professional callousness, negligence, and sheer incompetence are age-old forms of malpractice. With the transformation of the doctor from an artisan exercising a skill on personally known individuals into a technician applying

scientific rules to classes of patients, malpractice acquired an anonymous, almost respectable status. What had formerly been considered an abuse of confidence and a moral fault can now be rationalized into the occasional breakdown of equipment and operators. In a complex technological hospital, negligence becomes 'random human error' or 'system breakdown', callousness becomes 'scientific detachment', and incompetence becomes "a lack of specialized equipment." The depersonalization of diagnosis and therapy has changed malpractice from an ethical into a technical problem." Illich

"The pain, dysfunction, disability, and anguish resulting from technical medical intervention now rival the morbidity due to traffic and industrial accidents and even war-related activities, and make the impact of medicine one of the most rapidly spreading epidemics of our time." Illich

Hence it is also of critical importance to 'Life Medicine' and the 'Life Doctor' to recognise not only the many ways in which 'The Illness is the Cure' but also the converse: how illness itself can result from or be exacerbated by their supposed biomedical 'cure', whether in the form of drugs or surgery, hospitalisation, poor doctor-patient communication – not to mention the anxiety and stress induced by the increasingly detached, dehumanising and depersonalised approach to patients by medical practitioners and in 'modern' healthcare institutions. This is made worse by what Michael Balint[2] called 'the collusion of anonymity' – the way patients are regularly bounced from one specialist to another with no-one ever taking responsibility for them as a person – and the norm of short, 6-10 minute consultations. Doctors claim that given their workload longer consultations would be quite impossible, ignoring the fact that the 'Long Consultation' practiced by Balint – particularly if also approached with a view to exploring connections between the patient's life history and problems and their medical history and symptoms

– would without doubt significantly reduce the number of appointments and consultations sought for or needed by patients and in this way actually reduce the workload of doctors. The Long Consultation – up to an hour or more – would also restore a rich, personal and human dimension to doctor-patient communication. In this way it would also boost the innate potential of doctor-patient communication to fulfill an intrinsically healing function itself.

In contrast, the type of disappointment, dissatisfaction, stress and anxiety so often induced in patients through sheer shortness of standard consultations – not to mention reducing the dangers of negligence, the depersonalized mode of doctor-patient communication and 'collusion of anonymity' that go with it – themselves innately iatrogenic. The 'Great Time Barrier' to consultations with physicians both mirrors and reinforces a major social dimension of iatrogenesis. This is a social culture of manic economic busy-ness in which people do not have or grant sufficient time to their own bodies and bodily self-awareness, in which health itself is defined purely economically – in terms of the individual's capacity for work and employment and in which Big Pharma promotes pills for any symptoms which interfere with their jobs – as if these symptoms were not in themselves a meaningful and important form of bodily rebellion against of lives dominated by anxieties and pressures surrounding jobs and employment. A social environment in which 'making a living' – living purely to earn money under any circumstances or conditions – dominates life itself is intrinsically pathological.

The biomedical model of illness buttresses and reinforces this social environment and its pathology, its principle being to get patients 'back on their feet' i.e. back into employment or wage slavery as quickly as possible, albeit at an essentially counter-productive cost to the health, not just of their bodies but of their lives as a whole – the social dimension of medical iatrogenesis.

As Illich notes:

"People would rebel against such an environment if medicine did not explain their biological disorientation as a defect in their health, rather than as a defect in the way of life which is imposed on them or which they impose on themselves."

His summary:

"A professional and physician-based health-care system that has grown beyond critical bounds is sickening for three reasons: it must produce clinical damage that outweighs its potential benefits; it cannot but enhance even as it obscures the political conditions that render society unhealthy; and it tends to expropriate the power of the individual to heal himself and shape his or her environment."

References:

[1] Starfield, Barbara MD MPH *Journal of the American Medical Association, 2000*
[2] Balint, Michael *The Doctor, His Patient and the Illness*

Making Things Worse
through Medication

(see also appendices 3 and 4)

"...serious reactions to prescription drugs are responsible for 250,000 Britons being hospitalised each year – with aspirin, diuretics, warfarin and NSAIDs (non-steroidal anti-inflammatory drugs arthritis the main offenders." Ben Ong

"The majority of the cancer patients in this country die because of chemotherapy, which does not cure breast, colon or lung cancer. This has been documented for over a decade and nevertheless doctors still utilize chemotherapy to fight these tumors." Allen Levin, MD, UCSF

"...at least 250,000 people have attempted suicide worldwide because of Prozac alone and that at least 25,000 have succeeded." Professor David Healy

Millions of prescriptions for highly profitable drugs are handed out each year by doctors – even though the 'clinical trials' which made them available often show them to be barely more effective than placebos. At the same time, sales of over-the-counter (OTC) drugs such as pain killers bring in equally huge profits – despite often leading to chronic dependency. The counter-productivity of their possible side effects (doing the very opposite of what they are prescribed for) and the often severe and chronic withdrawal symptoms generated by different classes of common legal drug medications is shown below – using information from the makers and users of these drugs, together with the 'small print' in the instructions and warnings to patients that come with them. Just as the price paid for drug medications is kept artificially high by clever marketing – so also does the price paid by the body for using them continue to rise.

Drug class: ANXIOLYTICS (a new name for tranquilisers)
Side effects and/or withdrawal symptoms – *addiction leading to acute and chronic anxiety, irritability and restlessness, panic attacks, seizures, chronic sleep difficulties and/or muscular tension*

Drug class: SLEEPING PILLS such as temazepam
Side effects and/or withdrawal symptoms: *chronic rebound insomnia, nightmares, premature deaths (up to 500,000 in the U.S. alone according to the British Medical Journal Open Journal).*

Drug class: ANTIDEPRESSANTS (SSRI-type such as Seroxat/Paxil/Prozac)
Side effects and/or withdrawal symptoms – *depressive or manic symptoms, suicidal thoughts, suicide, aggressive behaviour, extreme violence*

Drug class: ANALGESICS (prescription or OTC pain killers and headache pills such as codeine or paracetemol)
Side effects and/or withdrawal symptoms – *nausea, digestive problems, chronic or recurrent rebound headaches.*

Drug class: ANTIINFLAMMATORY drugs such as Ibuprofen used for conditions such as arthritis
Side effects: doubling the risk of strokes and miscarriage.

Drug class: ANTICONVULSANTS (for epilepsy, nerve pain and seizures)
Side effects or withdrawal symptoms – *seizures*

Drug class: ANTIBIOTICS (for bacterial infections)
Side effects and/or withdrawal symptoms: *increased susceptibility to infection from increasingly resistant bacteria*

Drug class: PRESCRIPTION SKIN CREAMS (for skin disorders or infections)
Side effects: *acute or chronic skin damage and disorders, infections or inflammations*

Drug class: STATINS (for reducing cholesterol and protecting from heart attacks & strokes)
Side effects: *muscle weakness, fatigue, heart attacks, shortness of breath or difficulty breathing, strokes and death*

Drug class: BIPHOSPHATE BONE DRUGS (for osteoporosis and brittle bones)
Side effects: *increased risk of bone fracture*

Drug class: DIET PILLS
Side effects: depression, suicidal ideation, suicide

Drug class: ANTI-SMOKING PILLS
Side effects: suicide, suicidal thoughts, depression, nausea and vomiting

Drug class: VACCINES
Side effects: *increased susceptibility to infection (for example to flu, measles, polio etc.)*

EXAMPLE: below is a list of side effects included in the maker's own patient information leaflet for a skin cream currently prescribed for skin infections, reddening, swelling and itchiness and a variety of other skin conditions and disorders.

LISTED SIDE EFFECTS: *Severe rash, burning and stinging feeling, skin irritation, itching skin, worsening of your eczema, thinning of the skin, small veins near the surface of the skin become visible, stretch marks, itchy rash and skin inflammation in the area where the medicine is used, red spotting rash around the mouth or chin, skin of the face may become puffy, irritation to the eye s and mucus membranes (such as lips or genital area).*

Biomedicine as
Money-Driven Medicine

The increasing trend toward the privatisation of medicine has its roots in the privatisation of illness *as such* – and in the massive corporate profits that can be derived therefrom.

Yet to reduce illness to the private property of an individual's body is to wholly ignore the role played in illness by the *sickness of the world and planet* they live in – whether in the form of economic deprivation, ecological destruction, environmental poisoning and – last but not least, worldwide wars.

Then again, endless political debates about how to deal with the ever-increasing costs of funding for national or private health provision all fail to get the central point – namely, that in capitalist economies, the medical diagnosis and treatment of illness is essentially *big business* and *money-driven* – exploited for the promotion of new medical drugs and technologies. That is why the big pharmaceutical companies make more profits than all the Fortune 500 corporations put together.

What is conventionally regarded as 'science-based' or 'evidence-based' medicine is actually *nothing of the sort* – given the corners cut by Big Pharma in testing new drugs, in informing the public on their true and often minimal efficacy, in warning them of their side-effects and often serious dangers – not to mention the massive sums of money spent *not* on costly 'R&D' but purely on marketing the latest drugs and treatments to doctors and surgeons. Even the most reputable medical professionals and 'experts' are now regularly paid to have articles offering misleading 'evidence' for the efficacy and 'safety' of new drugs and medical technologies published in their name – whether or not they have participated in that research or even so much as read the articles sent for their signature. In reality, modern medicine and its treatments have been acknowledged by the *Journal of the American Medical Association* itself to be *the third leading cause of death* after cancer and diabetes.

Money-driven medicine has effectively turned patients themselves into commodities for sale by their physicians – offering a source of profit not just through drugs but through expensive hi-tech testing and 'treatment' technologies. All this at massive expense to national health services and/or to the profit of private health providers milking health insurance companies or even public health services.

The truth is that illness is essentially big business, that 'Big Pharma is Big Bucks and Bad Medicine', and that today's 'evidence-based' medicine is essentially Money-Driven Medicine . Indeed any drug or new medical technology that actually 'cured' a disease would be fatal for the profits of the entire Medical-Industrial Complex. Nevertheless the *promise* of cure is constantly promoted by this multi-trillion dollar medical industry – one with vast lobbying power and almost complete monetary control of regulatory organisations such as the Food and Drug Administration in the U.S.A.

"The pharmaceutical companies have become the favourite whipping boy in discussions about the corrupting influence of money in medicine. And the companies deserve a lot of the criticism they receive ... but I want to be clear that they are not the only problem. The larger truth is that creating new patients and making more diagnoses benefits an entire medical-industrial complex that includes Pharma but also manufacturers of medical devices and diagnostic technologies, freestanding diagnostic centers, surgical centers, and even academic medical centers."

Dr. H. Gilbert Welch *Over-Diagnosed – making people sick in the pursuit of health*

To put it bluntly, there are surely understandable *reasons* for people feeling or even getting seriously anxious, depressed or sick if they can't earn a living wage, can't rent or pay for housing, if their homes are threatened with foreclosure, if they face a daily threat of joblessness – or can see no chance of realising their life potentials. Yet modern 'scientific' medicine consistently ignores such reasons for both mental and physical illnesses, instead reducing them to a result of chemical imbalances in the brain or biological 'causes' of one sort or another. In this way it totally denies all *life-meaning* to illness – and its relation to the innate sickness and sickness-generating effects of capitalism itself.

Complementary medicine and proponents of alternative psychosomatic, psychoanalytic and existential understandings of illness frequently either ignore or downplay its social, political and economic dimensions. For capitalism also profits from illness in another way – by manufacturing it on an industrial scale through the dis-ease generated by what Marx called wage-slavery. This is the prostitution of the individuals' 'labour power' i.e. their bodies – to make profits for an employer, only for the employee to be casually disposed of through unemployment at times of economic downturn.

Yet what 'employment' itself means in capitalism is that anyone from skilled and experienced workers, to unemployed graduates, budding artists, musicians or scientists whose education or training, skills, interests and actual *work* has no current 'market value' can be forced into employment in the form of any low-paid job offered to them, even if it doesn't pay them a minimum or living wage – or in no way actually 'employs' their true skills, gifts or potentials.

In these circumstances, illness can thus serve as a form of *mute political protest* at the economic demands imposed by capitalism and the distress this imposes on people. For it offers the individual time to temporarily reclaim their body as their own, and allow it to embody and symbolically register their felt dis-ease and distress in what, for most, is the only socially acceptable way – through medical disease symptoms. The problem is then that their bodies are immediately *reclaimed* by medical professionals and the medical-industrial complex, in a way that actively furthers the process of translating and transforming an individual's felt 'dis-ease' into some medically diagnosable 'disease'. The patient's body is perceived and treated as a biological machine – rather than as a living embodiment of the human being. And as with any other machine, the aim is to repair it and restore its economic functionality.

For just as capitalism identifies work solely with 'employment' that profits an employer, so also it identifies 'health' solely with an individual's economic 'functionality', i.e. the capacity for 'employment' in the labour market rather than the capacity to engage in personally meaningful activity or work – irrespective of its 'market value'. Similarly capitalism recognises as 'illness' only that which interferes with the mechanical functioning of body and mind in the performance of mechanical tasks, physical or mental. All this has recently become ever clearer through governments making receipt of welfare benefits for the dependent on tests designed only to show that (totally irrespective of the individual's medical condition and indeed even if they are terminally ill) they are still capable of *employment of some sort* – even if they can't get a job, even if that job does not pay a living wage and even if it is clearly *damaging* to both their medical health and their essential 'health' i.e. their capacity for living a meaningful and fulfilled *life*.

The role of the doctor in what is ever-more evidently a money-driven medicine is – paradoxically – to rule out entirely from consideration the larger life context in which an illness first manifests – not least its economic context and the effect of the latter on the patient's social world and relationships. Thus, loss of housing, jobs or life opportunities of the sort that lead to disheartenment and loss of heart on the part of patients count for nothing – until and unless this loss of heart manifests as diagnosable symptoms of 'heart disease '. These are then, like all other forms of illness, cold-heartedly treated as if they had nothing to do with the patient's actual life whatsoever. The role of the biomedical doctor is principally to act and do – to *treat* patients and not to talk with them – and certainly not to *listen* to them, to hear and feel their inner 'dis-ease' and learn about the health of their *lives* and relationships. The seemingly idealistic aim of improving patients' health and 'saving' or 'extending' patients' lives through medical tests and treatments of all sorts is pursued at any cost to their bodies as a result of serious side-effects and at whatever expense to their real health i.e. their *quality* of life.

The result is a veritable epidemic of 'preventative' screening – at high cost to public health services – but resulting in over-diagnosis and over-treatment, even of people with no symptoms whatsoever. This leads in turn to widespread 'iatrogenetic' (medically caused) illnesses – which then require yet further medical treatments. A prime example is screening men for prostate cancer by conducting blood tests which measure their level of 'PSA' (Prostate Specific Antigen). If this is found to be above a set figure, intrusive biopsies are then regularly conducted. These can produce the very symptoms of prostate cancer they were supposed to prevent from emerging – as well as increasing the likelihood of any actual cancer spreading through the body. Yet as many doctors admit, most men die *with* and not *from* prostate cancer – whereas surgical and drug treatments for it can and often do dramatically reduce their quality of life, for example through making them impotent or incontinent.

Constant government, media and press propaganda regarding 'health risks' of all sorts, together with mass screening programs, serve a vital role in maintaining money-driven medicine and the medical-industrial complex – creating a type of mass hypochondria which feeds it with new patients to be medically processed or peddled with new drugs. No better was this pathological state of affairs expressed than by Illich:

"People who are angered, sickened and impaired by their industrial labour and leisure can escape only into a life under medical supervision and are thereby seduced or disqualified from political struggle for a healthier world."

Illich, Ivan *Medical Nemesis, The Expropriation of Health*

(see appendix 7)

The Focus of Biological Medicine –
The Clinical Body

The focus of biological medicine is the 'clinical body'. This clinical body is not the actual body of any individual human being – not my body or yours. Instead it is a body constituted entirely by a *body of knowledge* – specifically the body of knowledge accumulated in the form of medical terms and textbooks and imparted through medical and clinical training. The 'gaze' of the physician derives entirely from this body of medical and clinical knowledge – and is directed only at the 'clinical body'. It is a purely *clinical gaze* – one which turns the body into an object of medical-scientific examination and clinical testing.

In his book *Medicine, Rationality and Experience*, medical anthropologist Byron J. Good describes how, in the course of medical training, the body is progressively depersonalised. In particular, through their training in anatomy and the dissection of corpses, medical students begin a process comparable to a type of extended and intense period of almost cult-like indoctrination –in the course of which they gradually cease to see a human body as that of a *person* – and cease also to see the *interior* of that person as a space of containing personal thoughts, feelings, memories, fears and desires etc. Instead the person's interior is reduced to the anatomical structures revealed by cutting through the body's surface.

"In normal reality, the body surfaces – the skin, the hands, the eyes, the face, the clothing convey personhood. The interior of the person is his or her thoughts, experiences, personality."

Interviewing a medical trainee, Good cites a student's own words to reveal how, in the anatomical laboratory "As the skin is drawn back a different 'interior' reveals itself:

"Emotionally, a leg has such a different meaning after you get the skin off. It doesn't mean at all what it meant before. And now the skin, which is our way of relating to people – I mean touching skin is ... getting close to people – how that is such a tiny part of what's going on, it's like the peel of an orange. And once you get that off you're in this whole other world."

Good remarks that "This whole other world" becomes the paramount reality in the anatomy lab.

He also reports that *"While participating in anatomy as an observer, I would occasionally be walking along a street and find myself a body amidst bodies, rather than a person amidst person. I found myself attending to anatomical features of bodies I passed, rather than perceiving them as persons with social characteristics or imagined lives. Students describe vivid experiences of this sort."*

Through its exclusive focus on diagnosing and treating the 'clinical body', neither the individual's *felt* body, the individual human *being* – nor the individual world of *meaning* in which they live – actually *have any place in biological medicine* at all. Consequently, biological medicine – no matter how much treatment it gives to the clinical body – *cannot actually 'cure' a single human being.* Instead only the patient's illness can do that – through recognition of its meaning for the patient *as* a human being.

Reference: Foucault, Michel *The Birth of the Clinic*

The Non-Existent Patient – chronic illness, cancer and the work of Arthur Kleinman

The terms 'existential medicine' or 'life medicine' as I also term it, have a very direct meaning in relation to what is taken as medicine today – biological medicine or 'biomedicine'. For the reality is that from the perspective of biomedicine the patient neither *exists* as a human being, nor is seen or understood as having any *life* beyond the life of his or her body. This is not a philosophical claim but one attested by countless patients' experience of the way they are treated by their physicians, i.e. precisely not treated as human beings with real lives and therefore effectively just treated as living corpses.

In the case of chronic illness, this paradox of the 'non-existent patient' is exacerbated by the way in which even the patient's lived bodily experience of illness – and of its daily effects on their lives – is something which physicians almost never acknowledge or take any interest in, let alone seem capable of showing the least bit of empathy for, clad as they are in the emotional armour of 'clinical distance' that has been drilled into them through their training as the only proper and 'professional' bearing to maintain – one which reduces both patient and illness to a mere anonymous 'case' to be 'managed'. It should not need emphasising what effects this very bearing has on the health of the patient, both physical and psychological, given the experiential, emotional and existential quarantine it places them in and the loneliness this creates. In contrast, no one has more articulately acknowledged or given more vivid examples of patients' daily lived experience of illness – not least chronic illness – than Arthur Kleinman has in his book entitled *The Illness Narrative – Suffering, Healing and the Human Condition.* Almost the *entire book* would need to be cited to do justice to it in this regard, so I must restrict myself to a selection of just a few sections from it:

"The undercurrent of chronic illness is like the volcano: it does not go away. It menaces. It erupts. It is out of control. One damned thing follows another. Confronting crises is only one part of the total picture. The rest is coming to grips with the mundaneness of worries over whether one can negotiate a curb, tolerate flowers without wheezing, make it to the bathroom quickly enough, eat breakfast without vomiting, keep the level of back pain low enough to get through the workday, sleep through the night, attempt sexual intercourse, make plans for a vacation, or just plain face up to the myriads of difficulties that make life feel burdened, uncomfortable, and all too often desperate. It has always seemed to me that there is a kind of quiet heroism that comes from meeting these problems and the sentiments they provoke, of getting through each day, of living through the long course with grace and spirit and even humor; sick persons and their families understand the courage, even if most others do not.

Chronic illness also means the loss of confidence in one's health and normal body processes. The asthmatic can no longer count on unobstructed breathing or a quick end to a fit of coughing. The epileptic lives under the very point of the sword of Damocles, uncertain when a fit will come. The sufferer of chronic sinusitis goes from partially blocked nasal passages on one side to some obstruction on both sides, then to completely stopped up nasal passages with fullness, pounding in the ears, and mouth breathing – which interferes with sleep and causes air swallowing and its effects (gas, abdominal cramps). The sick person intervenes with nasal inhalers or oral decongestants. The former are transiently useful, but over time have less effect and may produce rebound sinus congestion. The latter may produce abdominal discomfort and lethargy, and they may worsen asthma. Each time the cycle of symptoms begins, the sufferer loses faith in the dependability and adaptability of basic bodily processes that the rest of us rely on as part of our general sense of well-being. This loss of confidence becomes grim expectations of the worst, and, in some, demoralization and hopelessness."

"For the chronically ill, details are all. To cope with chronic illness means to routinely scan minute bodily processes. Attention is vigilantly focused, sometimes hour by hour, to the specifics of circumstances and events that could be potential sources of worsening. There is a daily quest for control of the known provoking agents. Enervating decisions must be made about when to initiate or terminate an activity, when to move from base line medication to second level drugs, and when to seek professional help. And all this occurs in the context of active lives that are filled with the same pressures, threats, vagaries, and exultations that make of normal living such a "blooming, buzzing confusion" (James [1890] 1981, 462). Is it any wonder that exhaustion is one of the common shared experiences of chronic illness?"

It is in the context of the patient's lived experience of illness, together with its effects on their lives and social relationships, that there arises what is all too often an almost wholly unseen or unheard need for psychological and psychosocial support and understanding – not least given the common experience that chronic illness, whether terminal or not, can often have a morbidly *demoralising* effect on the patient's relation to *life as such* – and even contribute to their premature death.

Kleinman again:

"...there is a controversial body of medical and anthropological literature on psychogenic, self-willed, and voodoo and magical deaths, which suggests that individuals can come to believe that they are socially dead – a belief shared by their social circle – and can die in a psychophysiological reaction. Engel (1968;1971), conducting research at the University of Rochester, has identified in patients with serious chronic illness a complex of "giving-up, given-up" that correlates with unexplained sudden death. Hacket and Weisman (1960; Weisman and Hacket 1961), working at Massachusetts General Hospital, found that surgical patients who strongly believed they would die in fact died much more frequently than other surgical patients ... In my experience, fear of dying ... is common among the chronically ill and their families. For many patients with chronic illness the fear comes as vague, amorphic ruminations that are crystallized when patients enter a terminal stage of their disorder or when there is a severe exacerbation of symptoms. It is important to remember that most patients with chronic illness do not have an acutely life-threatening problem and that many, perhaps most, will not die of their chronic illness. Indeed, there is an old saying among clinicians to the effect that nothing is as effective at teaching a person how to live a long life as the experience of chronic illness. For some patients, convictions of dying or giving up are not delusional perceptions of their current situation, but rather perhaps early premonitions and remarkably sensitive recognitions of mortal, though subliminal, bodily changes. In the gray zone of serious but not life-threatening chronic illness, such perceptions may be accurate reflections of extraordinary psychophysiological sensibility. For most, however, such a sixth sense responds to emotional reactions, personality type, life situation, and even cultural background (for example, Jews have been shown to be more fearful of symptoms and the threat of death than Old Yankees) (Zborowski 1969; Zola 1966). If there is a single dimension of illness that can teach us something valuable for our own lives, then it must be how to confront and respond to the fact that we will all die ... There is no better example of what I mean than the sick person's coming to terms with death."

The patient's experience of *demoralisation* – not just through illness itself but through empathic failure on the part of physicians, lends great appropriateness to Kleinman 's use of the term *Remoralisation* to suggest the aim of a wholly new type of "medical psychotherapy" – akin to what I call Life Medicine. By 'medical psychotherapy' he did not mean any standard or standardised form of therapy – and certainly not psychiatric treatment of a sort which *pathologises* a patient's possibly quite morbid or death-preoccupied psychical states – but rather a type of therapy which instead recognises patients' needs for psychological understanding and psychosocial support as something no less and in some ways even *more* important to their health, both psychological *and* physical, than any form of biomedical care and treatment (which is anyway usually given in clinical settings wholly alien to and separate from the intimate context of the patient's own personal life – therefore further *alienating* the patient from that life). However, as Kleinman writes on 'Remoralisation':

"Instilling or rekindling hope in the chronically ill patient (and often in the family, too) is an essential, though poorly charted, clinical domain. Of course, there are models of short-term psychotherapy. But these have not been widely translated into the care of the chronically medically ill (for an exception, see Karasu and Steinmuller 1978)... Care for the psychological needs of the chronically medically ill is a field with few markers, like those unexplored portions of the maps of ancient times that carried the ominous warning, "From here on dragons!"

The fact that even short-term counselling of any sort is usually only given as a form of 'palliative care' to those patients seen as terminally ill, i.e. on a fast-track to *death*, symbolises a complete failure to recognise and respond to the psychological dimension of illness as such – and chronic illness in particular – in a patient's *life*, and that quite irrespective of however long or short that life may turn out to be. Indeed, from the perspective of Life Medicine, it may be hypothesised that illnesses becomes 'chronic' precisely through the persistent – chronic – failure to offer the types of 'medical psychotherapy' that I call 'Life Doctoring'.

Another symbol of this failure is the way in which diagnoses of *cancer* in particular have become so culturally charged with morbid connotations. It is as if one particular type of disease has become artificially singled out *as* a symbol for the way in which illness *in general* can come to gradually 'colonise' – to invade and pervade – ever more areas of a patient's *life* – doing so in the same way that cancer cells can come to 'metastasise' to colonise different parts or organs of a patient's body. This symbolism would also explain the disproportionate amount of money spent on 'cancer research' – as well as on expensive but largely ineffective and often life *damaging* forms of cancer treatment. It is as if the 'C'-word has, in Freudian terms come to both 'condense' and 'displace' important dimensions of illness *as such* – which continue to go almost wholly unrecognised in their significance, having to do with both the patient's lived experience of illness and with the personal, social, economic and cultural life contexts in which it both arises and is experienced.

In highlighting such contexts, Kleinman offers a stark account of how a poor black female patient (Mrs. Flowers) suffering from a whole range of intense worries and *life pressures* is reduced in her clinician's cursory medical report to a mere case of chronic hypertension, i.e. high *blood* pressure – one for which the 'cure' is simply medications and a reduction in salt intake. Kleinman 's transcript of a consultation between this patient and her physician (Dr. Richards) shows the latter's obsessive focus on the purely bodily dimension of her condition as opposed to its life dimensions – and his complete failure to register the most obvious temporal and symbolic links between them – even when these are made quite explicit by the patient herself (and underlined in the sections from the transcript I cite below) as well as impatiently interrupting any talk about pressures in her life before she can even begin to say more about them. Kleinman introduces the transcript by describing the patient as a human being with a life outside the consulting room: being a mother of five, periodically unemployed but now working as a poorly paid waitress, having a partially paralysed mother, an unemployed pregnant daughter with a history of drug problems, a brother in prison whom she is afraid will also get involved with drugs, his 12-year old daughter who has problems of truancy and minor delinquency and, last but not least, a 'friend' she refers to – Eddie Johnson – in reality, her long time male companion, recently killed in a barroom brawl.

Some extracts from Kleinman 's transcript:

Dr. Richards: You said you had headaches?

Mrs. Flowers: Sometimes I think my life is one big headache. These here ain't been too bad. I've had 'em for a long time, years. But in recent weeks they been badder than before. You see, a year ago last Sunday, Eddie Johnson, my friend, you know, Uh huh, well, he died. And....

Dr Richards (interrupting): Are the headaches in the same place as before?

Mrs. Flowers: Yeah, same place, same feelin', on'y more often. But you see Eddie Johnson had always told me not to bother about...

Dr. Richards (interrupting again and changing the subject): Have you any difficulty with your vision?

Mrs. Flowers: No.

Dr. Richards: Any other problems?

Mrs. Flowers: My sleep ain't too good, doc. I think it's because...

Dr. Richards (interrupting again...): Is it trouble getting to sleep?

Mrs. Flowers: Yeah, and gettin' up real early in the mornin'. I been dreamin' about Eddie Johnson. Doin' a lot of rememberin' and cryin'. I been feelin' real lonely.

Dr. Richards: Any other problems? *I mean bodily problems?*

Mrs. Flowers: No, 'cept for tired feelin, but that's been there for years. Dr Richards, you think worryin' and missin' somebody can give you headaches?

Dr. Richards: I don't know. If they are tension headaches, it might. But you haven't had other problems like dizziness, weakness, fatigue?

Mrs. Flowers: That's what I'm sayin! The tired feelin', it's been there some time. And the pressure makes it worse. But I wanted to ask you about worries. I got me a mess o' worries! And I been feelin' all down, as if I just couldn't handle any more...

Dr. Richards: ... Right now why don't we do a physical exam and see how you're doing?

Mrs. Flowers: I ain't doin' well. Even I can tell you that. There's too much pressure and it's makin' *my pressure* bad.

Dr. Richards: Well, we'll soon see how things are going.

Mrs. Flowers spells out the connection she clearly senses between pressures in her life that are getting too much for her and "my pressure" – her diagnosed hypertension. Dr. Richards clearly does not. Hence in his medical record Mrs. Flowers all but ceases to *exist* as a human being and reduces the worries and pressures in her *life* to a set of numbers. I cite from Kleinman 's record of this medical record:

39 year-old black female with hypertension on hydrochlorothiazide 100 mgs. daily and aldoment 2 grams daily. Blood pressure now 160/105. Has been 170-80/110-120 for several months, alternating with 150/95 when taking meds. Has evidence of mild congestive heart failure. No other problems.

"No other problems." One can hardly think of a phrase that, in the context of this far from untypical medical record, more blatantly exposes the complete separation between *the life of the human body* and the life of the *human being* that lies at the very foundation of biological medicine.

Note: though biomedicine has, since Kleinman wrote his book, grudgingly come to realise the relation between 'stress' and hypertension, this has led to words such as 'stress' and 'stressor' becoming loose 'umbrella terms' – as a result of which *they too* grant permission to ignore the *highly individual nature and m*eaning of events and circumstances affecting the health of specific patients and calling for recognition from physicians.

The Failure of Biomedicine
to Explain Pain

One of the most common and important aspects of illness that biological medicine can't explain is *pain*. The standard biomedical model of pain is called *nociception* and deals with the neurons that 'detect' pain, which are termed 'nociceptors'. This term is relatively new – in the past one spoke of 'pain receptors'. This term was abandoned because of its all too obvious questionability. For how can neurons 'receive' or respond to pain 'signals', when pain as such is essentially a *subjective experience*. So instead of pain receptors neurologists speak now of nociceptors, a term derived from the Latin *noci* (meaning 'hurt') and emphasise that what these receptors 'detect' is not actually pain as we experience it in real life, i.e. subjectively, but actual or potential *injury* or *damage* to external or internal tissue and organs.

As for how the actual subjective experience of pain comes about, this is explained by the nociceptors transmitting signals to the brain via the spinal column. The brain then responds by 'allowing' or 'producing' a subjective experience of pain. Yet how the brain can 'produce' a subjective experience *of any sort* – in this case pain – is left unexplained by this 'explanation'. Instead, the pseudo-explanation implicit in the old idea of 'pain receptors' is simply reversed, i.e. rather than having to explain how a neuron can detect a subjective experience such as pain, what is now left unexplained is how it can *create* such an experience as a result of tissue damage - particularly given that biology regards bodily tissue itself as basically *insentient*. The result is that biomedicine now claims that the true 'source' of pain is neither localised nerve receptors – nor is it wherever you *actually feel pain in your body* – but lies precisely where you *don't and cannot feel it* – in the brain. Thus the pain you actually feel in your toe after stubbing it, for example, is, according to this model, nothing but a *subjective illusion or sensory hallucination* created by the brain through a neural mechanism. This standard biomedical 'explanation' of pain is maintained despite the fact that:

1. It is counter-intuitive, running contrary to our lived experience of the source and site of pain.

2. It offers no explanation at all of how the brain can produce a subjective experience of pain.

3. It is premised on the idea that pain is a consequence of physical injury or damage, and so cannot explain why, for example: *"...about 65% of soldiers who are severely wounded in battle and 20% ... report feeling little or no pain for hours or days."*

4. It does not explain why *"...no apparent injury can be detected in 70% of people who suffer from chronic low back pain..."*[1].

5. It does not explain why even the most acute of pains can spontaneously arise and then subside without *any identifiable physiological change occurring*.

6. It does not explain why hypnosis and acupuncture can alleviate or even completely eliminate pain without any pharmaceutical or surgical intervention – even to the point of facilitating entirely *pain-free surgery* without any use of anaesthetics.

7. It does not explain acute, chronic or recurring symptoms of muscle pain (myalgia) or nerve pain (neuralgia) for example in the form of fibromyalgia, or of facial and trigeminal neuralgia – where there is often no evidence of damage to muscle tissue or to the nerves or nerve sheaths.

8. It does not explain many forms of common pain – for example particular types of headache with no clearly identifiable physical cause. Seeing them as a result of 'stress' does not explain why someone leading a generally stressfully life should experience just one particular type of pain (or any other illness symptom) or why they do so at a particular time or times and not others

9. It does not explain the experience of 'phantom pain' – pain experienced in the region of amputated limbs where there are no longer any neural pain 'receptors' or 'nociceptors'.

Points 3 and 7 present just a few of *many examples* in which – contrary to and in a way wholly unexplained by the standard neurological theories of pain – either injury occurs *without pain* or pain is experienced *without injury*.

Just as biomedicine seeks to 'explain' illness without first of all asking or seeking to 'explicate' what 'illness' or 'disease' essentially *is*, so also does it seek to 'explain' pain without first of all asking the most basic question of all – what essentially *is* 'pain'? Yet as Martin Heidegger points out:

"All explanation reaches only so far as the explication of that which is to be explained..." [my stress]

So: *"What good is all explaining if what has to be explained remains unclear?"*[2]

Pain is a perfect example of the *basic philosophical quandary* of biomedicine as such – namely the failure of all its explanations of illness to address and incorporate its lived, subjective dimension, and the chicken-egg question this gives rise to: namely is the felt *subjective* experience of 'dis-ease' (of 'feeling ill') a mere effect of 'being ill' – of having some 'objective' physiological disease or disorder? Or could it be that it is the other way round? This is the essential question that is avoided in biomedical explanations of pain. For whereas in ordinary language we speak of 'painful' life experiences or of feeling emotionally 'pained', 'wounded' or 'hurt', biomedical science discards this everyday *language of life* for neurological terminologies and explanations which seek to reduce pain to an effect of purely 'physical' or 'physiological' phenomena – yet without any explanation of how the *subjective* experience of pain arises from them. Indeed simply by turning the pain into an *object* of scientific or medical explanations, biomedicine implicitly *rules out in advance* any attempt to explicate the essentially *subjective* character of pain and instead turns this into a mere 'secondary' phenomenon arising from purely 'objective' neurological mechanisms.

"The idea of one basis for science and another for life is from the very outset a lie." Karl Marx

By simply shunting off both painful life experiences and 'emotional pain' into a second and entirely *separate life domain* from bodily pain, the biomedical explanation of pain is classically *dualistic* – not just separating 'mind and body', the 'psychic' and the 'physical', but also and above all separating *life itself* from what is claimed to be a true account (*logos*) or 'science' of life (Greek *bios*) – namely what is called 'biology'. Then again, by turning pain into an *object* of biological and neurological explanation however, not only does biomedicine entirely fail to explain its subjective essence, it also 'shoots itself in the foot' when it comes to *treating* pain – so-called 'pain control' or 'pain management'. For not only doctors but also patients tend to turn their own subjective pain into an *object* – into something they 'have'. This is unfortunate for the patient, because the bearability of pain and our capacity to live with it depends principally on our capacity to *be the pain* we experience rather than experiencing as some thing or 'object' affecting us.

'Being the pain' – *becoming it* – is the most effective way to stop experiencing it as some sort of bodily entity or object *separate* from our self and therefore 'causing' us to *suffer* in a way over which we actually have *no control* at all *except* through medication. Instead it allows us to identify with the pure *awareness* of pain – an awareness which is *not itself* anything painful. Indeed, actively choosing to *intensify* our awareness of pain – even the most acute pain – can, paradoxically, alleviate pain suffering – as well as releasing insights into its source in our lives (see Case Example 1).

From the perspective of Life Medicine, pain is first and foremost an experience of the subjectively experienced or 'lived' body and not the so-called 'physical' body or any of its organs, not least the brain. For if the assumptions of 'brain science' itself are followed to their logical conclusion, what we perceive from the outside as the human physical body and its internal organs – including the shape and form of the brain itself – is ultimately but a subjective perceptual 'phantasm' constructed and projected outwards *by* the brain. This is the sort of philosophical *reductio ad absurdum* to which, as Heidegger indicated, 'reductionist' brain science ultimately leads – both in general and in relation to pain. For taken to its ultimate conclusion we end up with a worldview in which there is nothing we perceive or experience that can count as real except the brain, even though, paradoxically, our very perception of that organ we call 'the brain' is, according to neurological models of perception itself, nothing but a construction of the brain. Despite these philosophical paradoxes we see an increasing flood of media propaganda for so-called 'brain science' – a science that identifies who we are as human beings with our brains is evidence for this – and a useful prop for manufacturers of brain-altering drugs, including what can be highly addictive analgesics or 'pain killers'. The term itself is an interesting one – akin to the term 'killer cells' or the notion of 'fighting illness'. In contrast we have the following words of Seth and of Ivan Illich taken from the appendices of this book.

"... pain and suffering are also obviously vital, living sensations – and therefore are a part of the body's repertoire of possible feelings and sensual experience. They are also a sign, therefore, of life's vitality, and are in themselves often responsible for a return to health when they act as learning communications." Seth (see appendix 6)

"A myriad virtues express the different aspects of fortitude that traditionally enabled people to recognize painful sensations as a challenge and to shape their own experience accordingly. Patience, forbearance, courage, resignation, self-control, perseverance, and meekness each express a different colouring of the responses with which pain sensations were accepted, transformed into the experience of suffering and endured. Duty, love, fascination, routines, prayer, and compassion were some of the means that enabled pain to be borne with dignity."

"The pupils of Hippocrates distinguished many kinds of disharmony, each of which caused its own type of pain...Pain might disappear in the process of healing, but this was certainly not the primary object of the ... treatment. The Greeks did not even think about enjoying happiness without taking pain in their stride ... The body had not yet been divorced from the soul, nor had sickness been divorced from pain. All words that indicated bodily pain were equally applicable to the suffering of the soul." Illich (see appendix 7)

To be sure, the use of 'pain-relieving', 'pain-killing' or analgesic drugs is a godsend for many people, though most of these (for example aspirin and opiate based drugs such as codeine or morphine) are not modern pharmaceutical inventions but based on natural plant remedies (willow bark or the poppy plant) which have been known about for millennia. Yet the effectiveness of such drugs in itself tells us nothing about the experience of pain, its effect on patients' lives – or its source in their lives. Pain may, of course, be a direct result of tissue and nerve damage, whether through inflammation, injury or surgery. Yet this does not explain the immense subjective variation in individual pain sensitivity and tolerance.

On the other hand, in the case of headache for example, pain, experienced bodily, may serve to quite literally 'bring to a head' painful emotional states and experiences. From the perspective of Life Medicine bodily pain in general almost invariably serves to *localise* in a more or less acute or chronic way what might otherwise be experienced as a more or less amorphous, unconscious and *non-local* sense of dis-ease connected with painful life events or experiences. Yet to suggest, as biomedicine does, that some experiences of pain are purely 'psychogenic' – implying that they are somehow subjectively 'imagined' by the patient just because they have no identifiable anatomical 'cause' – is to deny the essentially subjective nature of *all* sensations of bodily pain, whether we 'explain' them biomedically – as produced by the brain – or not.

The complete failure of biomedicine to explain the nature of pain is perhaps one reason why, apart from pain specialists, physicians in general tend to be rather disinterested in the patient's subjective experience of pain – except as a sign or symptom of disease they can objectively identify or diagnose. It also explains why in medical literature relating to different forms of surgical procedure, one almost never finds so much as *a single mention* of how patients *themselves* actually feel after their surgery – even on such a basic level of how much pain they experience and for how long. Thus an operative procedure may, in biomedical terms, be deemed entirely 'successful' even if a patient experiences intense pain for weeks, months or even years following surgery – thus totally ignoring the *damage* that pain itself (and other side effects of biomedical intervention) can inflict on a patient's *life*. That is not to say that pain killers will not be liberally prescribed – yet this too is often done without a thought for or mention of their own side effects or addictive properties.

All this fits uneasily with the Hippocratic oath of 'Do no harm'. In all too many cases, this harm actually begins with the very first consultation with a biomedical physician, if, as is so often the case, the physician completely fails to hear and empathise with the emotional pain which the patient is, in so many cases, simply seeking an attentive and empathic ear for. To find that a physician has 'no time' – in all senses of this term – for any subjective or emotional dimension of the patient's communication having to do with their life outside the consulting room is a form of empathic failure the experience of which is *in itself* a painful and harmful one. Yet it was only thanks to the pioneering work of Michael Balint [3] – now rarely recalled, recognised or applied – that doctors were introduced to the idea that not only their own clinical training but also their own *personal psychological defences* may play a crucial role in leading them to completely *block or filter out* any element of a patient's communication that might touch a raw or painful emotional 'nerve' *in their own life and psyche.*

Such expressions as 'touching a raw nerve', 'feeling hurt', or speaking, for example, of a life event or experience as having been 'painful' or 'excruciating' – far from being merely metaphorical, show us how the everyday language of *life* offers us a better guide to the essence of pain *as such* – as *pain* – than any biomedical 'explanations' of it as some purely bodily and neurological process. For such explanations, as we have seen, actually explain nothing about the experience of pain – and in effect reduce it to a sensory hallucination conjured up by the brain – thus making nonsense of 'scientific' distinctions between 'real' pain on the one hand and so-called 'phantom' pain or 'psychogenic' pain on the other. Nor do such explanations help us understand many cultural and religious phenomenon, for example how a torturer may be compensating for an inability to feel their own emotional pain by inflicting physical pain on another, or why in certain cultures, ritually self-inflicted pain is not seen merely as some of form of penitential act or 'self-harm' but is understood instead as a medium of mystical religious experiencing – connecting the worshipper to the pain of a revered martyr or even that of God himself. Finally current explanations of pain fail to explain the well-attested ability of yogins and fakirs to experience neither bleeding nor any pain at all even whilst piercing their own flesh – or how the use of acupuncture has been proved capable of preventing any experience of pain during surgery, thus eliminating the need for either local or general anaesthetics.

More importantly however, biomedical and physiological approaches to bodily pain deny it any intrinsic *meaning* or healing purpose. Yet pain can serve many important healing purposes besides 'nociception' – registering actual or potential tissue damage.

Examples:

- Allowing painful life experiences and emotional pain – 'inner pain' – to be experienced in a more intense bodily way and brought to a focus through painful bodily sensations.

- Allowing an otherwise only vague or dimly experienced sense of dis-ease in one's life to become more sharply and more acutely felt through the experience of bodily pain.

- Allowing the individual to express and elicit an indirect empathic response to their otherwise *unrecognised or unfelt* inner pain – their 'inner scream' – through such expressions of physical pain as grimacing and groaning, writhing of the body or 'screaming with pain'.

- Allowing the individual to obtain temporary relief from their inner pain through conventional forms of bodily pain relief.

All these purposes of pain serve to prevent not just the human body but the *human being* from suffering on-going or further 'damage'. Conversely, even where pain *is* related to actual tissue damage, this may be because it is the only way the individual is currently able to more fully experience, express and communicate their inner emotional or existential pain. This is also the reason why some individuals do engage in intentional and conscious self-harm – seeking a temporary sense of release from their inner pain through creating sensations of physical pain. On the other hand, a period of acute physical pain may also occur *after* the painful life issues behind it have been resolved – offering a sense of final cathartic release from them.

As a result of its failure to explain pain, the most important question *never* asked by biomedicine is whether the experience of pain can be approached as a form of healing *meditation* – rather than simply just as a sign of something 'wrong' or an object of pharmaceutical *medication*. So the idea that a form of 'pain therapy' may lie in consciously choosing to *identify* with or even *intensify* sensations of bodily pain – to give them *more attention and awareness* rather than less – is never for a moment considered – even though it is in this way alone that we may come to deeper insights into those painful aspects of our lives (and not just our bodies) the experience of bodily pain may itself *be an awareness of.*

Worse still, if there is no recognition on the part of biomedical physicians for the emotional pain people experience in their lives, who knows just how many times *morphine* eventually becomes necessary as a substitute for the *empathy* that is both craved by and denied to patients – and that long before their inner, emotional pain or 'life pain' finds expression as bodily pain.

References:

1.   Melzack and Wall, *The Challenge of Pain*, Hardmondsworth: Penguin Books, 1982

2.   Heidegger, Martin *Zollikon Seminars,* Northwestern University Press, 2001

3.   Balint, Michael *The Doctor, His Patient and the Illness* Churchill Livingstone, 1957.

Example: a brief case of headache

A patient complained about having a bad headache at the beginning of a session with her therapist and just before she was about to go on holiday with her partner. Asked when the headache had started she reported having woken up feeling fine but then worrying about the holiday. This was because she had promised her partner not to take any work-related books with her, knowing he was afraid that reading them would preoccupy her for too much of their time together.

However, whilst packing before the session she had realised that she really would like to take at least a couple of her books along with her – but also felt bound by the promise she had made to her partner not to do so. In other words it was the inner pain, fear and guilt about a desire whose result might be to hurt her partner that triggered the headache.

When her therapist suggested that she might resolve this relational dilemma by indeed taking a couple of books with her – but at the same time resolving not to get lost in reading them at the expense of spending time with her partner – she immediately realised that this could indeed offer a practical way of *reconciling* her desire not to hurt or cause pain to her partner with her equally sincere wish to enjoy at least some time reading her books. When she came to a decision in the session to follow this suggestion and to also share and negotiate a new compromise and new promise with her partner she became aware that her headache had totally disappeared.

Biomedicine as a Religion
of Salvation from Sickness

"Science *is* the new religion." Nowhere, outside perhaps cosmology, is this saying by Martin Heidegger more evident than in the field of biomedical science, which, like a religion, claims an absolute monopoly on true 'knowledge' in matters relating to illness and the human body – regarding all other or earlier forms of medicine as based on primitive or pre-scientific 'beliefs' in contrast to true biological 'knowledge' in the form of biomedical 'science' – the 'one true faith'.

The cultural kinship between biological medicine and religion goes even further and deeper however. To begin with, the words 'whole', 'hail', 'hale', 'heal' and 'holy' share a common origin. Hence the unhealthy is also the 'unholy', as echoed in the German word 'Unheil'. It is not surprising then, that some religions have therefore traditionally associated sickness with sin, not least Christianity – which also laid emphasis on the healing powers of Christ as part of his salvational role.

The theme of this chapter is that biomedicine effectively offers the same type of salvation as a religion, so that even whilst its emphasis is on salvation from sickness rather than from sin, nevertheless in today's health-obsessed culture, health as such has become a synonym of what is 'good' whereas illness is regarded as something not only intrinsically 'bad' but also associated with 'unhealthy' (read 'sinful') activities such as 'bad' foods, smoking, overeating, not taking enough exercise etc.

Thus it was only a small step from the demonization of *smoking* to the demonization and ostracization of *smokers* – who are constantly reminded by medical propaganda and gruesome images on cigarette packets that they will pay the price for their filthy habit or 'sin' – for example through eventually contracting one or another form of serious lung or heart disease as a form of punishment.

Biomedical science is not only a religion of salvation from the implicit 'evil' of illness but also and in this way a search for salvation from death itself. Indeed through advances in genetics, biomedical science holds out the ultimate prospect of overcoming death itself – through a form of physical immortality.

"Through the medicalization of death, healthcare has become a monolithic world religion." Ivan Illich

The new religion has evolved to the point of having its own Bible and Book of Genesis – namely the human genome – a bible which is understood by the medical-scientific high priests of this religion as literally holding *all* the keys to life and death, sickness and health – yet which only those high priests can decode and master.

Through this new bible the long-standing quasi-religious quest for 'miracle cures' on the part of biomedical science continues. For though medical researchers regularly complain about the exaggeration of such cures on the part of the media, pharmaceutical companies still promote their pills as 'magic bullets' with miraculous powers – and that however negligible their effectiveness in comparison to placebos, or however mysterious their mechanism of action is to biomedical science itself.

Nevertheless, as Illich also points out: "Public fascination with high-technology care and death…" continues, and can be understood, as the expression "…of a deep-seated need for the engineering of miracles."

A case in point is 'intensive care', which Illich describes "...as but the culmination of public worship organised around a medical priesthood struggling against death."

On the other hand, he also points out significant differences between the religion of biomedicine and the approach of traditional religions to illness and suffering.

"The major religions reinforce resignation to misfortune and offer a rationale, a style and a community setting in which suffering can become a dignified performance." The difference also lies in the different modes of interpretation of illness that these religions offer, whether "...as karma accumulated through past incarnations, as an invitation to Islam, the surrender to God; or as an opportunity for closer association with the Saviour on the Cross."

In contrast:

"Medical procedures turn into *black magic* when, instead of mobilising his self-healing powers, they transform the sick man into a limp and mystified voyeur of his own treatment." They also "turn into *sick religion* when they are performed as rituals that focus the entire expectation of the sick on science and its functionaries instead of encouraging them to seek a poetic interpretation of their predicament or find an admirable example in some person – long dead or next door – who learned to suffer."

Illich himself became a supreme embodiment of such an "admirable example" during the last ten years of his life, during which he refused hi-tech biomedical treatment for a painful and disfiguring facial cancer on the grounds that it would prevent him from engaging in the most innately fulfilling and therefore most essentially healthy dimension of his life – namely his work.

Yet as he also observed, the religious dimension of biomedicine is nowhere better exemplified than by the money poured into hi-tech cancer research and treatment, which increases in direct proportion to the ineffectiveness of such treatment – or its iatrogenic effects in either triggering or worsening cancer conditions as well as severely damaging the patient's quality of life (for example through carcinogenic chemo- or radiotherapy) and all this on the pretext of saving that life.

This paradox can only be accounted for by recognising that "Paradoxically, the more attention is focussed on the technical mastery of disease, the larger becomes the symbolic and non-technical function performed by medical technology ... Not only white coats, masks, antiseptics, and ambulance sirens but entire branches of medicine continue to be financed because they have been invested with non-technical, usually symbolic power."

This would also explain why entirely fake operations relying only on the symbolically suggestive power of mysterious forms of technology and belief in the god-like power of clinicians or surgeons have been shown, like placebos, to be capable of producing exactly the same results as real operations – with operating theatres serving as the innermost holy sanctum of hospitals – the *temples* of biomedicine.

This is not to say that emergency-room operating theatres and intensive care units do not and have not saved lives or that they should be abolished. But intensive hospital care for the 'terminally ill' is a different matter entirely – for as Illich notes, evidence suggests it does not increase life expectancy at all and in many cases it actually reduces it in comparison with *home care* – which allows the patient to "avoid the exile, loneliness and indignities which, in all but exceptional hospitals, await them." Thus "...patients who have suffered cardiac infarction themselves tend to express a preference for home care; they are frightened by the hospital, and in a crisis would rather be close to people they know. Careful statistical findings have confirmed their intuition: the higher mortality rate of those benefited by mechanical care in the hospitals is usually ascribed to fright."

'Putting the fear of God' – and of death – into patients is a more recent and one of the most perversely religious dimensions of biomedicine. Thus the current standard of what is bizarrely understood as 'ethical' practice on the part of biomedical clinicians is to present patients diagnosed with terminal illness with a *worst case scenario* as regards their maximum life-expectancy.

Thus a patient may be told that he or she has *at most* one year or less to live, even though the clinician well knows from experience and empirical evidence that though this *may* be the case, there can be absolutely no 'scientific' certainty in this respect – and that the patient may in fact live on for anything up for an indefinite number of years – or even, as also happen, go into remission.

The profound and stressful psychological impact of such prognoses – and that not just on the patient's state of mind but on their body – goes without saying. As a result it can prove tantamount to a self-fulfilling prophecy – a form of 'death by prognosis' – akin to a doomsaying religious prophecy or a witchdoctor's curse.

Just as religion has its own temples so does biomedicine – the hospital or clinical surgery. These are truly clinical temples, unadorned, like Lutheran churches, and replacing uncomfortable pews with cheap plastic chairs. Stands or shelves abound in every waiting room, replete with glossy printed religious tracts warning of the evils of this or that disease and/or of the price to be paid by unhealthy (read 'sinful') lifestyles.

The institutional hierarchy of biomedicine is also like that of a church, except that its bishops are managerial bureaucrats who preach the gospel of cost-cutting and the sanctity of efficiency. Consultation with the patients are ritualised time-limited 'procedures' which severely restrict the patient's ability to share their own lived experience of illness and its effects on their lives – something which anyway counts for nothing to the clinician unless the patient's own words can be immediately translated into the dry liturgical language and terminology of biomedical science.

The physician is not there to listen, understand and empathise but, like the dogmatic mouthpiece of a religious belief system – simply to *prescribe* what the patient must do – whether this means taking a pill or undergoing a further standardised 'procedure' whether in the form of a blood test, a scan, an operation or a further tightly time controlled consultation with a 'specialist' in one or other area of biomedical theory and practice. All such procedures are of course documented in the form of medical records, reports, test results and communications. The result is that the patient is ultimately reduced to a set of documented, biomedically framed accounts of their illness in which all traces of the patient's experience of illness have been purged.

As for the written 'prescriptions' with which patients regularly leave their clinic or hospital, these are comparable to the so-called 'indulgences' granted (or even sold) by the Catholic church, "proving relief from the temporal punishment resulting from the effect of sin" – or in this case sickness.

Finally, we should not forget also the religious and globally 'crusading' role of biomedicine in seeking to displace local, culturally and ethnically rooted understandings of illness – which, again, are seen as mere systems of 'beliefs' in contrast to the supposedly universal truth of biomedical 'knowledge'. Here we see something akin to the historical appropriation of local 'pagan' gods and symbols by Christianity. Yet if traditional local remedies can be displaced by – or, as is increasingly the case – modified and repackaged as *patented pharmaceutical products*, then of course this crusade also reaps big profits for Big Pharma – just as the Crusades were as much about bringing home booty as imposing new beliefs.

Illness as Deviance

"In Latin norma means 'square', the carpenter's square. Until the 1830's the English word normal meant standing at a right angle to the ground. During the 1840s it came to mean conformity to a common type. In 1880s, in America it came to mean the usual state or condition not only of things but of people... [It] was first given a medical connotation around 1840 by August Comte ... During the last decade of the nineteenth century, the norms and standards of the hospital became fundamental criteria for diagnosis and therapy. For this to happen ... it was sufficient that disease as deviance from a clinical standard make medical intervention legitimate... "

Ivan Illich, *Medical Nemesis, the Expropriation of Health*

Though they may or may not think very deeply about what is wrong with the social and economic system they live in, most people who suffer from being stuck in poverty, poor housing or boring, low-pay jobs would not think of asking what is wrong with *them*. Nor do people who suffer from the experience of war, floods or other natural catastrophes, deaths in their family etc. Yet when it comes to suffering experienced in the form of bodily symptoms of 'illness', then, unless their condition is clearly related to their immediate environment or living conditions (for example starvation, lack of clean water, radioactive emissions etc.) the first question people tend to ask themselves is 'What's wrong with ME?'

The question itself carries several implications. Firstly, the word 'wrong' implies that something abnormal and unnatural is going on in their bodies, i.e. a *deviation* from some *norm* of 'healthy' bodily functioning. Secondly, the question implicitly asks for a 'cause' of the body's deviant behaviour – and usually seeks an answer in the form of some medically diagnosable 'illness' or 'disease'. Indeed the sufferer might already be asking themselves speculative diagnostic questions such as 'Am I getting a cold?' or 'Might I have cancer?'.

A third, even worse implication is suggested by the little word 'me' – the implication of it being that not just a person's 'mind' or 'body' but *they themselves* are 'deviant' in some way. The belief that illness is a form of deviant bodily state or even deviant behaviour may be reinforced by feelings of shame or anxiety around it – for example, shame or anxiety about calling in sick and taking a day or more off work.

Such feelings are further reinforced if, as was revealed in a recent documentary on working conditions and regulations in Amazon warehouses – employees are actually given a 'black point' for simply taking half a day off work due to illness – or even just *feeling tired* at the end of a gruelling 10- hour night shift – and thus not fulfilling their pre-set performance targets. Worse still, the Amazon rule was 'three strikes' (three black points) and you're out – quite literally out of a job – and that quite irrespective of whether your symptoms (for example a bad or even chronically injured back) might actually *be due* to the excessive strain placed upon your body by the job itself (for example from having to constantly push heavy trolleys). In the case of Amazon, we must include also the mental stress of having the maximum time in which you are expected to pick up another item for the trolley literally *counted down in seconds* on a hand-held monitor carried by every employee).

This is but a particularly extreme example of how the very *phenomenon* that we call 'illness' is never itself brought into question. Is a worker's 'illness' merely their bad back, or some other psychological stress or physical strain symptom? Is it enough to have a doctor diagnose the patient's symptoms (for example as tendonitis or a damaged vertebra) to know what's 'wrong' – to know what the 'illness' is? Or is what is *really* 'wrong' the fact that institutionalised biological medicine limits the very phenomenon of illness to the patient's body and mind – failing to look for let alone 'diagnose' anything fundamentally 'wrong', 'ill' or 'sick' in their *life world*.

This narrow biomedical concept of 'illness' as a phenomenon is particularly obvious in the case of so-called 'mental illness' – where a person may for example, be medically labelled as suffering from a 'psychiatric disorder' called 'depression' – yet without taking into account any of the countless entirely good and valid *reasons* a person might have for feeling depressed, even severely or 'clinically' depressed (for example the actual or looming death of a spouse, loss of a home or job etc.). More broadly still (and though it seems almost a too blindingly obvious question to even ask, though it rarely *is* asked) what sort of medical 'mindset' is it that regards 'depression', 'cancer' and even 'Post Traumatic Stress Disorder' as 'illnesses' – but not exploitative *wage-slavery* or *war* – not even dropping atom bombs on whole populations or using carcinogenic uranium tipped bullets? Similarly, what sort of medical mindset is it that regards liver cirrhosis as an 'illness' – but not the mass marketing of alcoholic drinks or a culture of binge-drinking? The list of possible examples here is endless, yet they all point to a *wholly artificial division* between the sickness of individuals and that of society as a whole and social relationships in general – including the doctor-patient relationship – a division maintained not just by medical practitioners but all too often by their patients as well.

From the first question ('What's wrong with me?') comes another: 'What can I do about it?'. This second question too, carries many hidden implications and presuppositions. One major presupposition is that if a person has discomforting symptoms of any sort, then the natural and obvious course of action is to seek to *get rid of them* – and to do so both as soon as possible and by any medical means available. The idea that an illness may be a *natural expression* or even a *healthy* response to fundamentally unhealthy ways of living and relating, to distressing life experiences – or to a fundamentally sick world – does not even enter the medical mindset shared by most doctors and patients alike. Instead it is as if the whole place of medicine in society is simply to eradicate the symptoms of a sick society by 'privatising' them – reducing them to a *personal condition of individuals* and one that can be diagnosed and treated independently of their larger social and relational context of emergence.

What Martin Buber said of so-called 'mental illness', namely that "sicknesses of the soul are sicknesses of relation" can therefore *just as well* be said of so-called 'physical illnesses' too – 'sicknesses of the body'. Indeed it may be argued that 'sicknesses of the body' are there precisely to express and make us aware of 'sicknesses of the soul'. For the human body is not just a more or less well-functioning biological machine but a living relational language of the human being. And just as 'body language' constitutes the major component of all human communication and relating, so also is 'bodily sensing' (Gendlin) our most important way of staying aware of how we are experiencing our lives and life world as a whole – being a type of sensitive *field awareness* of that world as opposed to the more focussed awareness we apply to everyday activities in it.

As Carlos Castaneda put it: "The body *is* an awareness." This is an understanding central to the very essence of what we call 'body' – a word whose oldest etymological meaning is simply 'to be aware' or 'be awake'. Quite simply, the body itself, being itself so intimately connected with the world around us, also is aware of and *knows* that world more deeply and intimately than the intellect alone. Yet we are faced with medical mindset that, whilst it claims a huge amount of intellectual knowledge *about* the body, at the same time totally *ignores or devalues* the body's own *knowing* – that sensitive knowing awareness which the body most essentially *is.*

A second presupposition of the 'What can I do about it?' question is (except in emergency situations or where simple remedies suffice) the belief that *anything needs to be 'done' at all.* For more often than not, when patients present physicians with symptoms, their principal motive – beside the basic infantile one of wanting a parent figure who will 'make it better' – is simply to seek acknowledgement or 'registration' of their discomfort or suffering by another human being and – through the official role of the doctor in society – by society at large. The patient may also, consciously or unconsciously, be seeking someone who will recognise the ways in which they feel not just ill-at-ease with their bodies but ill-at-ease with their *lives*, i.e. recognition of the existential or life *dis-ease* that their body is communicating through their symptoms.

This is not the same thing as asking for a medically recognised 'disease' to be diagnosed. For though this is something which may be a comfort for some, for most patients diagnostic testing and its results often constitutes a further step on the road of separating their body from their being, their 'illness' from their *life* – including their life history, relationships, circumstances and conditions, dilemmas and 'dis-ease'. Taking this step may also lead to suggestions for medical treatment which only serve to reinforce this separation of illness and life, and which often also carry with them another presupposition latent in the question 'What can I do about it?'. This is the presupposition that if nothing is done about it, 'it' can or will only get *worse.*

On one level, we all have a tendency to respond to any form of bodily suffering in a basically infantile way – feeling upset by it, wanting it to go away immediately or seeking someone or something that will 'make' it go away – make us 'better' as soon as possible. We may also believe that if nothing is done the symptoms will either persist for ever or get worse in ways that are a further source of fear. This belief and the fear associated with it is often actively intensified by physicians (usually out of their *own fear* of negligence in ignoring the possibility of some serious or even life-threatening disease developing if what *may be* its first signs are not looked at more closely or its still harmless first stages not treated promptly). Indeed we could go so far as to say that the mindset of biological medicine is based on a fundamentally *paranoid* relation to the human body and bodily states. Thus the often amorphous sense of 'not feeling ourselves' that is often taken as the first sign of 'illness' may already alienate us from our bodies – leading us to experience them in a paranoid way as alien or persecutory bodies, altering and threatening the usual bodily sense of *self* we take for granted.

In today's medicalised world however, any suggestion that we might overcome this sense of alienation from our bodies in the way that human beings used to do for millennia – *by accepting and patiently bearing the discomforts, pain or incapacity we are suffering* – is regarded as a dangerous form of defeatism in the on-going medical 'war' against disease, i.e. against whatever genes, cells or microorganisms are currently held by medical 'science' to be the alien disease 'entities' responsible for that suffering. The role of the physician then, is reduced to one of merely identifying this alien entity as precisely as possible in medical terms, and then medically exterminating or surgically excising it. Hence instead of exercising the art of *patience* in the face of suffering people become willing 'patients', often colluding with physicians in a common war against the supposedly alien entities inhabiting their bodies. The biological fact that there are, all the time, *millions of times* more bacteria than cells in a 'healthy' human body (including pathogenic ones) is quietly ignored – as are many proven medical and biological facts that fly in the face of biological medicine.

104

The fact of the matter is also that in industrialised societies billions of people – even if *not* 'ill' in medical terms – are *already* unhealthily alienated from their bodies. They are so simply by virtue of having to sell their bodies' physical and mental capacities to an employer – for them to use or abuse at will for in the pursuit of commercial and corporate profit. Yet instead of this fact – this 'sickness of relation' – being taken as an illness in itself it is meekly accepted as an unalterable economic 'given'.

After all, we all have to 'earn a living', even if we have no option but to do so through what Marx described so well as "the alienation of labour" – a big part of which was the alienation of the labourer from his or her own body. The result is that 'health' *as such* has increasingly come to be defined as mere 'fitness for work', i.e. the capacity to 'function' economically and in this way conform to and sustain an economic system based on wage-slavery.

That the *human body* should rebel against this type of alienation and slavery through symptoms of 'illness' – even and particularly if as *human beings* we do not ourselves rebel – is surely a *healthy* response (and that even and particularly if it incapacitates or disables the individual's capacity to merely function economically as a 'healthy' corporate wage-slave).

And yet the *pseudo-religious dogma and moralistic judgement* that illness implies something 'wrong' with the body – or even with the person who is deemed 'ill' – stubbornly persists, thereby providing an on-going justification for the increasing medicalisation – and commercially highly lucrative *medication* – of almost every form of human suffering. Thus despite the no less commercialised proliferation of 'alternative' forms of medicine the *true alternative* to biological medicine finds almost no voice in our society. This is the alternative of understanding the very phenomenon of 'illness' in a way that transcends the boundaries of the body, of seeking and finding *meaning* in illness rather than seeking medical cures for it. By this I mean understanding what we call illness as something with an innately *healing* function – not something in need of cure or elimination but there to *cure us* – to free us from intrinsically unhealthy ways of thinking, relating, living and 'making a living'. Hence the provocative title of my book – 'The Illness is the Cure'.

One fundamental way in which each of us can therefore begin to alter our whole understanding of and relation to illness from this new and radical perspective is therefore precisely *not* to ask ourselves the sort of questions referred to at the beginning of this essay- questions such as what is 'wrong' with us or with our bodies. Instead we can ask ourselves what it is that our bodies are telling us is wrong with our *lives*. Similarly, instead of asking ourselves what we can 'do' to cure our symptoms we can ask ourselves what our bodies themselves are urging – or even forcing us – to start or stop doing *in and with those lives* (by which I do not mean things like stopping smoking or starting on the latest health tips and fads).

It is the reduction of *life* as such (Greek *bios*) in all its dimensions to the life of the body, and the reduction too of life's own meaningful 'speech' (*bios logos*) to a single science called 'biology' that together constitute the most basic falsehoods on which modern 'biological' medicine is built – preying on our need for instant fixes for any form of suffering.

Therefore a second way of fundamentally changing our relationship to illness is, like the Stoics and Pyrrhonian skeptics of ancient Greece, to refuse to *judge* any particular way of experiencing our body – and with it our minds – as 'better' than any other. This means also breaking with the conventional association of health with *happiness*. For it might well be that by fully accepting a bodily state of suffering associated with 'illness', not only do we not cease to be capable of happiness, but might actually experience a new and deeper state of 'happiness' or 'well-being' – one wholly *independent* of the presence or absence of 'illness' or suffering in our lives.

What we are speaking of is a depth of contact with our own innermost being (Greek *daimon*) that in and of itself constitutes a state of 'well-being' – one that the Greeks called *eudaimonia*.

On Life Medicine

Basic Principles of Life Medicine

- Illnesses have life *meanings* and not just biological 'causes'.

- People die *through* illnesses – not 'because' of them – and that only if they are *ready* to die.

- It is not illnesses that are the problem in our lives - but the *life problems* that express themselves as illnesses.

- The body is not a biological machine or a product of our genes but a living biological *language* of the human being.

- Health is not merely our capacity to 'function' economically in the labour market but an expression of the degree of fulfilment we experience in our lives, work and relationships.

Life Medicine is 'holistic' medicine in the truest sense, exploring the relation between the life of our bodies and our lives and life world as a whole.

Life Medicine challenges the whole separation between what is called 'physical ', 'organic' or 'somatic' illness on the one hand and 'psychological' or 'mental' illness on the other.

Life Medicine is not merely 'psychosomatic' medicine – it does not merely focus on a limited category of so-called 'psychosomatic' or 'stress-related' illnesses.

Life Medicine recognises that every bodily state is at the same time a 'psychological' state or state of consciousness – and that every state of consciousness is at the same time a felt bodily state.

Life Medicine recognises that for many if not most people, illness is the only way they can give expression to and gain recognition of the ways they are *ill-at-ease* with their lives.

Life Medicine affirms the healing value of illness itself, recognising that the sense of 'not feeling ourselves' that marks the onset of symptoms can be the beginning of a journey that leads to 'feeling another self' – one that feels more at ease with ourselves and our lives.

Life Medicine understands illness as a form of pregnancy with its own gestation period and labour pains. From this perspective, illness is not just something to 'bear' or put up with. Instead its purpose – one that Life Doctoring can help to fulfil – is to help us to give birth to and embody a new bodily sense of self and a new inner bearing toward our lives and life relationships. In this sense, it can be said that *the illness is there to cure the patient* – to offer them healing insights into themselves and bring about a healing transformation in their lives.

The Healing Value of Illness

"...the body's symptoms are not necessarily pathological, that is, they are not just sicknesses which must be healed, repressed or cured. Symptoms are potentially meaningful and purposeful conditions. They could be the beginning of fantastic phases of life, or they could bring one amazingly close to the centre of existence. They can also be a trip into another world, as well as a royal road into the development of the personality."

Arnold Mindell

"If people become ill, it is quite fashionable to say that the immunity system has temporarily failed – yet the body itself knows that certain 'dis-eases' are healthy reactions. The body does not recognise diseases as diseases in usually understood terms. It regards all activity as experience, as a momentary condition of life, as a balancing situation."

from *The Way Toward Health* by Jane Roberts (see appendix 6)

In its 'war' against disease – a war conducted at whatever cost to the state or to the individual – neither the meaning of illness nor the potentially healing value of illness are acknowledged by biological and genetic medicine. Life Medicine, on the other hand is founded on the recognition that illnesses can themselves serve many different healing purposes:

- Giving bodily expression to a felt 'dis-ease' – to ways in which we may feel ill-at-ease with ourselves, other people or different aspects of our lives.
- Forcing us to take 'time out' from merely 'functioning' in a physically or economically desired way.

- Helping us to feel, focus on and confront painful life problems – even if only through the way in which physical pain can itself focus the mind.
- Bringing us to a necessary 'crisis' in the root sense of the word – a decisive 'turning point' in our lives.
- Allowing us to fully express and reveal intense emotional pain by feeling and expressing it as a reaction to physical pain.
- Incapacitating us in a way that allows us to accept real limits to our capacities – limits we might otherwise have sought (or been put under pressure) to deny and overcome.
- Letting us become dependent on others in a socially acceptable way, and in this way to express dependency needs which we might otherwise think are unacceptable.
- Enabling us to indirectly ask for and receive emotional care and attention from others through the care of our bodies and being taken care of as 'patients'.
- Helping us to give more time and be more patient with ourselves and others by becoming 'a patient'.
- Providing a temporary respite from life problems by becoming a medical 'patient' in need of treatment and care.
- Providing a temporary but coherent organising principle for a person's life – built around their symptoms or around timetables of rest and treatment.
- Overcoming isolation and offering a medium of human contact through relationships with physicians or through the social environment of a hospital ward.
- Putting us into an altered state of consciousness – one in which we can come to feel ourselves and see our lives in a different way.
- Stopping us from just living in our heads and minds and helping us feel our bodies again – thereby giving us a fuller, more embodied sense of self.

- Transforming our 'body identity' and 'body speech' – bringing about and giving birth to a new bodily sense of who we are and new bodily ways of relating to others.
- Allowing us to identify with and feel close to an important person in our lives – living or deceased – who may have suffered symptoms of illnesses similar to our own.
- Giving symbolic expression to a subjectively felt *dis-ease.* For example heart conditions as a metaphorical expression of either 'loss of heart' or 'heartlessness', 'cold-heartedness' or 'faint-heartedness' etc.
- Giving birth to a new bodily sense of self or 'body identity' – one more in tune with one's current life, able to relate in new ways to others and respond in new ways to one's life world.

Finally, we must not forget the importance of illness as a quite natural way of dying or as a way out of intolerable life circumstances such as extreme poverty or war. The 'war' that biological medicine wages on disease on the other hand, is part of a wholly unnatural and wholly unwinnable war against the basic *life* realities of both aging and *death*. That is why people seek cosmetic or herbal 'elixirs' of youth and science seeks to develop bio-technologies that offer a purely physical form of immortality. What this reveals is a social culture that values quantitative longevity over quality of life, and why biomedicine uses all possible means – even the most toxic – to extend the lives of patients by mere months – at whatever economic cost and at whatever cost to a patient's *quality of life.*

Healing through Feeling

'Diagnosis' in Life Medicine and Life Doctoring does not mean seeking a medical label or 'cause' for one's symptoms. It means getting to know oneself in a new and intimate feeling way (*gnosis*) through (*dia*) one's symptoms.

Illness symptoms not only 'affect' one's life and one's overall mental, emotional or somatic state. Instead every bodily state or condition in other words, including states of illness – even a minor cold or flu – is not just some 'physical' state but *is* always and at the same time a *state of consciousness* – and vice versa. It is also a 'self state' or 'body identity' – imbuing us with a different sense not just of 'how' we feel but of *who we are*. That is why through giving ourselves time to simply feel our symptoms *more* intensely rather than less – we can come to experience illness in a new way – not simply as a sign of some possible 'disease' but as a way of experiencing ourselves – as a distinct state of consciousness and a distinct self state and sense of self, a different 'body identity'.

The key to self-healing is to feel and sense the symptoms we experience in a new way – not just as localised physical sensations or mental-emotional states however, but as self-states – as ways of feeling oneself and one's life. Any symptoms, if fully felt and followed in this way – meditated rather than medicated – will lead inevitably to healing insights into one's life and to a renewed and transformed sense of self. This is not because we are 'curing' ourselves without biomedical treatment, but because it is our very existence – our relation to life – that is what is most essentially calling for healing.

As in the 'Process-Oriented' work of Arnold Mindell, 'healing' can take the form of actively encouraging the patient to amplify or 'aggravate' their felt sensations of pain or discomfort – to feel them more intensely or acutely rather than less. What Mindell found was that this could bring about the release of emotions, mental images and inner comprehensions that expressed the felt meaning of their symptoms. Mindell has applied this method to all types of symptoms, and to all dimensions of the patient's experience of illness – mental, emotional and somatic.

If a patient fears or wishes for death for example, he might ask them, there and then, to die – thus encouraging them to fearlessly feel and face the 'death process'. He understood also that for some patients, as in essence it is for all of us, death itself is nothing to be fought against in principle – as biological medicine does – but it is an intrinsic part of *life* and is invariably a healing in itself i.e. a way of finding life meaning and fulfilment in other dimensions of reality in ways that might be or have become impossible in an individual's physical life and existence.

Like Life Medicine, Mindell's work challenges the historic and hitherto unquestioned premise of all forms of medicine – the fundamental belief that its purpose is to treat and if possible 'cure' disease and thereby also to prolong *physical* life and the life of the *physical body*. Ideas of a 'life after death' are considered to be a mere matter of personal 'belief' rather than a scientific question – not surprisingly given that current 'science' ignores the fact that the 'soul' itself has its own innate bodily form, and that our felt body, as a *body of awareness*, is indeed also an eternal 'soul body' which, like our dream body, has its source and reality in other dimensions of awareness beyond the 'physical'. Indeed Mindell speaks of what I term the felt body or 'lived body' – in other words our eternal *soul body* or *body of awareness* – as the 'dreambody' or 'dreaming body'.

This is a significant term for another reason. For it reflects also a deep comprehension that illness and its symptoms emerge in the same way as *dreams and their symbols* do and that illnesses can in this way be understood as 'body dreams' – or 'body nightmares'. From this point of view it makes no more sense to regard sickness as an 'unnatural' deviation from a 'normal' state of health than it does to regard dreaming as an unnatural or abnormal disruption of sleep, or to regard nightmares in particular as an 'unhealthy type' of dream. The biomedical model of illness on the other hand, based as it is on the premise that illness is a *meaningless* deviation from health, is as outdated as certain pre-Freudian 'scientific' beliefs that dreams are *meaningless* discharges of neurological energy.

Life Medicine, on the other hand does not see dreams as a mere function or by-product of some organ of the physical body such as the brain. Instead, as we have seen, it understands the so-called 'physical' body as but an externally perceived portion of our lived body as a whole – our soul. This is essentially a subjective body or body of feeling awareness – and one whose field of awareness transcends the boundaries of the flesh to embrace our entire life world and everything we experience within it. It is *this* 'soul body' that we also experience directly both in our dreams and after death. It expresses itself in and as our entire waking and dream environment. The terms 'dream body' or 'dreaming body' thus points to a fundamental truth – namely that we do not first 'have' a physical body – one which we then come to feel and experience subjectively and through which we experience a world – but rather *dream* our perception of the waking world and *body* a portion of ourselves within it in the same way that we do in the dream world itself.

Yet in broader terms, neither consciousness nor the body are something 'in' the world. Instead both worlds and bodies exist *within* consciousness, our entire experienced or lived world itself being itself our larger body or 'lived body'.

This body is composed essentially of patterned tones and qualities of *feeling awareness* which both *body* and *dream* themselves into different worlds and dimensions of our lived experience.

Dreaming on the one hand, and what Heidegger called *bodying* on the other, are thus intimately connected. In dreaming we *body* our feeling awareness in non-physical forms. Conversely, in waking life we 'dream' that feeling awareness into what then appears from the outside as our human physical form. Yet our 'felt body' – our subjective feeling awareness of this 'physical' body is in reality a *distinct body of awareness in its own right* – a 'soul body' that we both manifest physically and also give manifold form to in our dreams. Hence the type of connections between dream symbols and physical symptoms that Freud was aware of and that revealed themselves in the following example of what Mindell calls 'healing through feeling' – a basic and innate capacity of our feeling awareness or 'soul' and *its* body.

Case Example 1

from *Working with the Dreaming Body* by Arnold Mindell:

"A patient with whom I was working was dying of stomach cancer. He was lying in the hospital bed, groaning and moaning in pain. Have you ever seen someone who is dying? It was really quite sad and terrifying. They flip quickly between trance states, ordinary consciousness and extreme pain. Once, when he was able to speak, he told me that the tumour in his stomach was unbearably painful. I had had an idea that we should focus on his proprioception, that is, his experience of the pain, so I told him that since he'd already been operated on unsuccessfully, we might try something new. He agreed, and so I suggested that he try to make the pain even worse.

He said he knew exactly how he could do that and told me that the pain felt like something in his stomach trying to break out. If he helped it break out, he said, the pain worsened. He lay on his back and started to increase the pressure in his stomach. He pushed his stomach out and kept pushing and pressing and exaggerating the pain until he felt as if he were going to explode. Suddenly, at the height of his pain, he said 'Oh, Arny, I just want to explode!' At that point he switched out of his body experience and began to talk to me. He told me that he needed to explode and asked if I would help him to do so. 'My problem', he said, 'is that I've never expressed myself sufficiently, and even when I do it's never enough.'

This problem is an ordinary, psychological problem that appears in many cases, but with him it became somatised and was pressing him now, urgently expressing itself in the form of a tumour. That was the end of our physical work together. He lay back and felt much better. Though he had been given only a short time to live and had been on the verge of death, his condition improved and he was discharged from the hospital. I went to see him afterwards very often, and every time he 'exploded' with me. He'd make noises, shout and scream, with absolutely no encouragement on my part.

... It was then also that I discovered the vital link between dreams and body symptoms. Shortly before he had entered the hospital, the patient dreamed that he an incurable disease and that the medicine for it was like a bomb. When I asked him about the bomb he made a very emotional sound and cried like a bomb dropping in the air, 'it goes up in the air and spins around sshhhss ... pfftfff.' At that moment I knew that the cancer was the bomb in his dream ... his body was literally exploding with pent-up expression. In this way his pain became his own medicine ...

In a flash I discovered that there must be something like a dreambody, an entity which is both dream and body at once ... The way I discovered the concept of the dreambody was through what I called amplification. I amplified my client's body, or proprioceptive experience and I amplified the exploding process which was mirrored in his dream."

Basic Guides to Self-Healing

1. Meditating Specific Symptoms

- Give yourself time to be aware of your immediate *bodily* sensations of any state of illness or dis-ease. Ask yourself and become more aware *of where and how* you feel your dis-ease in your body.

- Remind yourself that the pure awareness of any sensation, emotion or thought – however painful – is *not itself* a sensation, emotion or thought, and is innately pain free.

- Staying aware of any localised sensation or symptom, remind yourself that it is itself *an awareness* of some aspect of your life-world and relationships that is a source of unease or 'dis-ease'.

- Wait until a spontaneous awareness arises of what specific aspect of your life-world it is that the sensation or feeling of dis-ease embodies – and is itself an awareness *of*.

- Grant awareness to one localised sensation or feeling of dis-ease or discomfort after another, staying with it long enough until it too recalls you to some specific aspect of your life world, present, past or future.

- Take time to follow this process through – making sure you attend to every region of your body *in* the process – until your *overall* sense of dis-ease lifts and your overall sense of self and body alters – transformed by the very awareness you are granting it.

2. Cultivating Whole-Body Awareness of Dis-ease

- Remember: only through awareness of your *body as a whole* can you gain and maintain a sense of your *self as a whole* – your 'soul'.

- When you feel ill therefore, do not focus solely on your symptoms – on localised sensations, thoughts or emotions – but instead seek to maintain a sense of your body, self and life *as whole.*

- If you feel yourself suffering from what you think of as a purely 'mental' or emotional state, remember that every such state is always accompanied by a particular *bodily* sense of yourself.

- Conversely therefore, even if your symptoms seem to be purely bodily, attend also to the thoughts and emotions that tend to accompany them – for these will give you the best clue to the underlying life-problem that they symbol ise.

- Understand too, that any mental, emotional and bodily state that you experience when you feel ill is at the same time a 'self state' or 'body identity' – a particular bodily way of feeling *yourself* – who you are.

- Attend therefore, not only to the way your symptoms 'make you feel' but to the way they make *you* feel – the overall sense of self or 'body identity' that accompanies them.

- If you can, *choose* to fully feel and indeed even amplify any felt sensations of dis-ease or sickness symptoms rather than seeking to suppress them.

- *Trust* that any mood or feeling, sense of dis-ease or bodily symptom – if it is given *enough time* to be fully felt, amplified and inwardly followed – will in time *automatically transform* itself into a new feeling, a new sense of your body and a new bodily sense of self or 'body identity' – one now free of the need to embody or 'somatise' itself through symptoms of one sort or another.

Note:

The lack of whole-body awareness *as such* in our generally mind and head-oriented culture is itself a type of basic social pathology – one that is not resolved through simply placing equal emphasis on the heart and emotions as well as on the head and intellect. For both thoughts and emotions are experienced in localised ways and in localised regions of the body. Authentic whole-body awareness on the other hand, is comparable to the awareness of one's body as whole – from top to toe, inside and outside – that is experienced in the womb, and that also arises when, for example, one enters and comes to rest in a hot bath. Maintaining whole body awareness means that this sensation of warmth pervading one's whole body – and maintaining one's awareness of it – persists unbroken, throughout the day. Put in other words the body as a whole – though having long left the warm and fluid waters of the womb – is itself experienced as a safe, fluid and warmth-filled womb of the self.

Illness as an Awareness

Every feeling, symptom, mental or physical state, together with our overall sense of self or 'self-state' is not just something we are aware *of*. Its meaning lies in the fact that *it is itself an awareness* of something. Thus a muscular tension, for example in the form of a tension headache, though we only be aware of it as a bodily tension, may itself embody an awareness of a particular tension in our lives, relationships or place of work.

Just as a person whose family has been made homeless or wiped out in a war has *good reasons* for feeling 'sick' or 'depressed', so do all feelings and symptoms have good reasons. They are not just programmed or mechanical physiological reactions to or 'effects' of external or internal 'causes'. Simply to label feelings as 'positive' or 'negative', to describe ourselves as 'well' or 'unwell', or to call the way we feel as 'good' or 'bad', is to deny the inherent *meaning* of all feelings – as an awareness of something beyond themselves. Symptoms of illness, like dream symbols, are a form of *condensed* awareness. Their *inherently* positive value and meaning lies in helping us to become more *directly* aware of what it is that they themselves *are* a condensed or embodied awareness of. Thus digestive problems are a condensed embodied awareness of an aspect of our lives or lived experience of the world we find difficult to 'stomach' or 'digest'.

Even though illness is often or mainly experienced through *localised* bodily symptoms (including 'mental' states such as a sense of confusion localised in our heads), every such symptom is also and always accompanied by a state of consciousness or 'mood' that pervades *our entire body* and in this way also affects our entire *bodily sense of self.* This bodily sense of self or 'self-state' is itself an undifferentiated *awareness* of what may be many different aspects of our overall *life world* that are difficult or uncomfortable, distressing or disturbing for us – thus giving rise to a general sense of 'dis-ease '. That is why, in order to find meaning in the overall bodily sense of 'unwellness' or 'dis-ease' that accompanies a specific illness, it is necessary first to experience it *as* a self-state. This means giving awareness to how any state of discomfort or dis-ease, however localised, imparts a specific overall tone, texture and colour to our subjectively felt body or 'lived body' *as a whole* – in this way lending also a specific tone and colour to our bodily sense of self or 'body identity' and to our experienced or lived *world* as a whole.

To pass from an experience of illness as 'not feeling ourselves' to one of 'feeling another self' – a distinct self or 'self-state' – means experiencing this distinct bodily sense of self. The 'other self' we experience through illness however is, by definition, *an experienced self* – a self we are aware *of.* Our self as a whole or 'soul' on the other hand, is not essentially any *experienced* self, symptom, state of consciousness or 'self-state', but rather the very *awareness* of experiencing it. To avoid becoming unconsciously identified with the self-states and symptoms of dis-ease, it is necessary to identify with that 'whole self' which is nothing *but* this awareness – the *experiencing self* rather than any *experienced self.* Only within the awareness that *is* this self – our 'awareness self' – can we in turn feel and affirm every particular feeling and self we experience or are aware *of.* We are as much aware of our *self as a whole* – our soul – as we are aware of our *body* as a whole. Yet the 'body' of our whole self or soul – our *awareness self* – is not just our physical body but *our entire life world.* For it is an awareness that embraces everything and 'every-body' in our world, from our immediate present reality and relationships to our past and future – and ultimately the entire universe.

126

The *second* step in healing ourselves through awareness is therefore to experience each and every localised bodily sensation or symptom, no matter how subtle, *as an awareness* of some specific aspect of our larger body – of our life world. Thus by giving more awareness to a localised muscular tension we can experience it *as* an awareness of a specific tension in our life world. Through a meditational process of giving awareness to each and every *localised* bodily feeling or sensation of dis-ease – no matter how subtle, and by making sure we attend to each and every *region* of our body in the process – we can come to experience each of these feelings and sensations *as* an awareness of some aspect of our larger body or life world. Through this process we are literally putting ourselves together – 're-membering' and making whole that larger body that is our life world *as a whole*. By simply *granting* awareness to each region of our bodies and each sensation or feeling of dis-ease or discomfort we experience within it, our overall sense of dis-ease and overall 'self-state' will automatically begin to alter. For we will feel ever-more pervaded, lightened and healed by that very self which is the *awareness* we grant to our overall self-state – our body, self and our life world *as a whole*.

Case Example 2
Two Ways of Responding to Symptoms

1. A personal secretary finds herself stuck in a job with a bullying and abusive boss. Fearing to express her feelings of irritation, anger and humiliation 'face to face' and 'face up to' her boss, feeling vulnerable in the face of the unpredictable rage this might unleash in her boss, and afraid with good reason that it might be 'rash' to risk her job by doing so, she keeps 'a straight face' in the face of all the bullying. Over time her feelings come to the surface in her body itself – in the form of an 'irritating' and 'angry' red skin rash. Lacking a way to 'face up to' her boss, let alone 'whack him one' – even though she is itching to do so – the rash appears on her face, arms and hands. Plagued by itching, she scratches and irritates her own skin until it blisters and bleeds – an activity that provides, unaware to herself, some satisfaction in releasing her 'bad blood' towards her boss. But her feelings of embarrassment and shame about not being able to face up to her boss become displaced by shame and embarrassment about the rash itself. So she goes to her doctor. Not even thinking that asking her questions about her life world might have any diagnostic significance, the doctor is therefore completely blind to the metaphorical *meaning* of her 'angry rash'. Adopting a conventional medical approach, the doctor's sole interest is in diagnosing the rash as some form of skin disorder and treating it – and prescribes a cortisone cream. The problem is that she then becomes dependent on the cream, which far from helping her to become tougher and more 'thick-skinned' emotionally, has the side-effect of thinning her actual skin surface itself, making it more vulnerable to embarrassing sores and bleeding. Eventually she feels forced to either lash out at her boss and risk being fired or else to leave her job voluntarily and seek another boss.

2. The same secretary allows herself to fully feel the emotions of anger, vulnerability, shame and humiliation she experiences. This means allowing herself to feel them fully in her body as a whole, neither repressing them nor being provoked to *rashly* reacting from them. She allows herself to *be* angry rather than 'getting angry'. She also reminds herself that the pure awareness of an emotion, however intense, is not itself an emotion or impulse but something innately emotion- and impulse-free. Letting herself *feel* and *be* angry makes her feel less vulnerable to her boss's bullying. Instead the anger transforms itself into an awareness of the bullying that allows her to see it for what it really is – as the expression of a deep insecurity and vulnerability in her boss himself. At the same time, by bearing her anger and feeling it fully in her body, it transforms into a sense of a different self within her, a self strong enough to face up to her boss – or to anyone – in a calm, non-hostile but nevertheless firm and resolute way. By *bodying* this new self through her body language and tone of voice she feels ever less vulnerable to her boss and instead becomes aware of the vulnerability behind his bullying. Sensing this, he finds it strangely more difficult to be as bullying towards her as before. For now it is *he* who is aware of feeling an insecure, vulnerable self behind his anger. Initially fearing this self, he first intensifies his abusive bullying, only to find it met by a calm, resolute and firmly toned response from the secretary. Not being able to provoke her into 'getting angry' the secretary is not fired. And being now capable of bodying her anger through a new inner bearing she no longer needs to 'somatise' it through an angry red facial rash, or fear being fired.

Illness as an Altered State of Consciousness

From the point of view of Life Medicine there is no need to scientifically find or prove causal links or relations between 'body and mind ', 'body and brain '. Instead it is a matter of recognising that every bodily state *is* a 'mental' state, but in a much broader sense than usually understood – being a state of consciousness that is experienced just as much in a bodily way as in our 'minds'.

No 'subjective' state or 'state of consciousness' is merely something enclosed or encapsulated in our heads, brains or minds. Conversely the body as such is not something we merely perceive or are merely aware of 'mentally' – as if it were some object we carry around with us. Instead the body itself is but a particular shape and dimension of subjective experiencing – one that completely transcends the whole body-mind, body-brain division. This is why the notion of the 'felt body ', 'lived body' or 'subjective body' is so central to Life Medicine – and to the new understanding of illness it brings. For this new understanding makes it impossible, in principle, to separate our lived experience of illness into two separate categories that we call 'mental' and 'physical'.

A basic principle of Life Medicine is that every *bodily state* is also a *state of consciousness* and vice versa. That is why the experience of any bodily state or condition, even a minor ailment such as a flu or cold goes together with a new and different state of consciousness – a state of consciousness that is not limited to one's head or mind but pervades one's entire body.

Conversely, different types of 'mental' or 'emotional' states are also states of consciousness not confined to the head or mind – but felt and experienced in a bodily way, for example as a particular sensation arising from a state of muscular tension in one's chest, stomach or guts.

"Every feeling is... a mood that embodies in this or that way."
Martin Heidegger

What we call a 'mood' however, is nothing we are simply mentally aware of in our heads, but is rather a particular tone and quality of embodied, feeling awareness – one which is always in one way embodied as different degrees and qualities of *muscle tone and tension* – which is why no state of 'mental' stress or tension is not at the same time a state of muscular tension.

"A mood makes manifest how one is..." Martin Heidegger

In other words, a mood is not just something purely mental but is a bodily way of *feeling ourselves*. This is reflected in the fact that the question *'How do you feel?'* is synonymous with the *question 'How are you?'* For the way we 'feel' is the way we 'are' – and vice versa.

For this reason however, any alteration or change in *how* we feel or are is at the same time a change in our sense of *who* we are or feel ourselves to be – a change in our identity or sense of self that is felt in an immediate bodily way. For in a most literal sense the 'you' that feels sick or tired is not the *same* 'you' that feels healthy, bright and alert.

Thus, not only is every *bodily state* also a *state of consciousness* – it could also be described as a 'self-state' or 'body identity'. For the way we feel our bodies cannot be separated from the way we feel ourselves. *How* we feel in our body affects not just our mind but *who* we feel ourselves to be – our 'bodily sense of self' or 'body identity'. That is why, when people begin to feel ill they might speak of 'not feeling themselves'. This basic 'dis-ease' of 'not feeling ourselves' is both the essence and first sign of illness – being not only an altered state of consciousness (how we feel) but also an alteration of our bodily sense of self or body identity – of *who* we feel ourselves to be.

The Immune System and Body Identity

In the framework of biomedicine 'body identity' is reduced to our genetic or *biological* identity and associated in particular with the immune system – which is seen as 'defending' our biological identity against threats and attacks from 'foreign bodies' in the form of pathogenic bacteria, viruses or mutant and cancerous cells, or any type of genetic material such as organ transplants that consist of 'non-self' cells (a term actually used in immunology).

Today more than ever, much fuss is made about 'health' being dependent on maintaining or restoring a strong 'immune system' or with strengthening the body's immune 'defences', which is why countless food products and supplements are advertised that claim to do so. On the other hand even biomedicine acknowledges that most discomforting or painful symptoms of illness (such as a runny nose or swelling and painful joints) arise from the activity of the body's immune system. Indeed many illnesses are recognised as resulting from an immune system that is too strongly defensive and as a result is *overactive* – leading to so-called 'autoimmune' diseases such as arthritis in which the body's immune 'defences' are used to attack its own cells. Alternatively, the body's immune system may be at such a high alert and so overactive and 'strong' for long periods that it ultimately weakens or collapses. Its very strength and activity therefore may ultimately result in precisely the sort of weakness that makes the body susceptible to infection and other types of illness.

In contrast to biomedicine, Life Medicine understands the strength of our immune system – the degree of immunity of our *bodies* – as an *embodiment* of the degree of immunity of our *self* or *identity*. Thus a *too rigid* or *strongly defended* identity or sense of self – one completely 'immune' to natural and healthy processes of *change* and adaptation to life – may find biological expression through an *over-defensive* and *over-active* immune system, which then actively seeks out threats to our biological identity that would otherwise be ignored or are ignored by the immune systems of other people. An over-rigid or immune *self* – or one that experiences deep *identity conflicts* – would explain many so-called 'auto-immune' disorders. A more healthily and naturally 'strong' identity or sense of self on the other hand would also explain what biomedical immunology can't explain – why some people 'catch' diseases which are supposed to be highly infectious whilst others don't – even from spouses or children they live with or during widespread epidemics. Nor can biomedical immunology explain why most of the bacteria, viruses and even damaged, mutated and 'cancerous' cells that biological medicine regards as 'causes' of diseases are all in fact *constantly present* in most healthy bodies.

Biomedicine simply takes it for granted that 'health' is the protection of a *fixed* biological and genetic identity – one 'immune' from all change. The problem with this theory is that it prevents biomedicine from coming up with any explanation of why it is that the immune system, though it may launch attacks on transplanted cells and tumours, does *not* launch attacks on a no less alien or foreign body that can grow within the human body – namely the baby growing in a pregnant mother's womb? And whilst biomedicine has effectively come to treat pregnancy and birth as something fraught with as many dangers as an illness, therefore requiring hospitalisation and the use of hi-tech medical equipment, the body itself clearly does not regard pregnancy as a disease or the baby as an alien or foreign body growing inside it – despite the differences in its DNA to that of the mother. Life Medicine, on the other hand, understands 'health' itself as a capacity to allow our body identity or sense of self to be altered and transformed in response to our life world and life experiences. That is why, instead of *treating pregnancy as if it were a type of illness*, Life Medicine understands *illness itself as a type of pregnancy* – the meaning and purpose of which is precisely to allow us to gestate and give birth to a new 'bodily sense of self' or 'body identity'. A key aspect of health, not as a mere state but as an on-going *life process* is therefore the capacity to pass from a state of 'not feeling ourselves' to one of 'feeling another self' – and of learning to embody or 'give birth' to that self through new and different ways of relating to our lives and life world.

Health and Illness as Life Processes

The different ways in which it is possible to interpret and respond to discomforting alterations in our bodily sense of self – in particular that bodily sense of 'not feeling ourselves' that accompanies even the most *minor* of symptoms such as feeling a cold or flu coming on – take us to the very heart of the contrast between Biomedicine and Life Medicine. They also enable us to understand both health and illness as self-states and *life processes* rather than merely as bodily states or biological processes.

A key aspect of both health *and* illness as *life processes* is how we interpret and respond to the essential 'dis-ease' of 'not feeling ourselves' – a dis-ease that may either precede or accompany discomforting symptoms of illness. One option is to feel this dis-ease and its symptoms merely as a *sign* of some biological disease or disorder – leading to what I call 'the illness process'. An alternative is to feel our dis-ease as a state or pregnancy and our bodily state as the womb of a new and different sense of self gestating within us – a self we do not need to 'defend' against or 'fight' with our body's immune system. This is what I call 'the health process' in contrast to 'the illness process', the stages of both of which are described below:

The Health Process

1. 'Feeling ourselves' in a familiar and 'normal' way that we identify with feeling 'healthy'.

2. 'Not feeling ourselves' – feeling a change in our bodily sense of self or body identity.

3. Choosing to actively affirm and identify with our altered bodily sense of self or 'body identity'.

4. Giving ourselves time to meditate our felt-disease in the context of our current lives.

5. Passing from 'not feeling ourselves' to 'feeling another self' – to experiencing the change in our bodily sense of self not as something that is 'not me' or 'other than self' but as a distinct self in its own right.

6. Seeking to actively embody and in this way give birth to the new sense of self that is pregnant in our dis-ease through new ways of being and relating to others and our life world.

The Illness Process

1. 'Feeling ourselves' in a familiar and 'normal' way that we identify with feeling 'healthy'.

2. 'Not feeling ourselves' – and experiencing this both as a felt sense of *dis-ease* and as the result of some 'thing' that is 'not self' or 'other than self'.

3. Identifying our felt dis-ease solely with some purely bodily state or illness symptom.

4. Seeing this symptom only as a sign of some 'thing' that is 'wrong' with us – such as a medically recognised 'disease'.

5. Seeking a medical diagnosis or 'cause' for our symptoms in some 'foreign body' such as a virus.

6. Seeking a 'cure' for our symptoms by some means of medically counteracting or cutting out that 'foreign body'.

The illness process is always culturally and linguistically shaped. Thus, whilst modern medicine might seek the cause of dis-ease in a foreign body such as a 'malignant' tumour or 'pathogenic' virus or bacterium, a witch-doctor or shaman might blame it on a malign spirit just as earliest Greek physicians blamed illnesses on 'ill-winds' or *pneuma.* Yet what *all* historical forms of medicine have tended to share in common is that any sense of 'not feeling ourselves' – rather than being taken as an opportunity to begin 'feeling another self' – is instead identified with feeling something wholly 'other than self' such as a foreign body or spirit, or a 'non-self' cell or organism. In this way however, the health process – passing from 'not feeling ourselves' to 'feeling another self' is *foreclosed* and gives way instead to the 'illness process'.

Illness as Pregnancy and
the Life Doctor as Midwife

If we understand illness in the framework of Life Medicine, i.e. as a life process comparable to gestation, then all forms of medical treatment or 'cure' are equivalent to an attempt to medically 'terminate' or 'abort' the new bodily sense of self or 'body identity' that is pregnant in the patient's dis-ease. Such premature medical termination or abortion of an illness has the immediate 'side effect' of preventing the patient from taking time to explore, understand and identify more clearly the new sense of self they are gestating and pregnant with – and to find ways of giving birth to it through a new way of living and relating. Abortive biomedical treatment may and does also frequently 'miscarry' in several others ways – not just through other side effects but also through actually intensifying the 'illness process' – the process by which a felt dis-ease is 'somatised' and as a result may take the form of ever more chronic or acute medical symptoms and diseases. Finally, even if a disease or its symptoms *are* cured – whether through conventional medicine, alternative medicine or 'spiritual' healing – if the underlying dis-ease behind it is not explored, the result may well be that the patient simply gives expression to this dis-ease through *other* symptoms or *another* disease – one that may be worse or more serious than the one supposedly 'cured'.

The 'health process' is a process of giving ourselves time to feel ourselves more deeply into a felt dis-ease with the aim of sensing it as an expression of a different bodily sense of self – rather than simply seeking to counteract or cure, suppress or exorcise its symptoms. Since so few people are able to approach any felt sense of dis-ease in this way however – through 'the health process' – this dis-ease may need to take the form of ever more acute or chronic disease symptoms for them to begin to do so. The illness process therefore, can also

138

provide a spur for the health process. Yet if, through the illness process, an individual's *dis-ease* has already reached the point of transforming itself into a serious biological disease, then some form of biomedical intervention may be unavoidable, if only to alleviate its symptoms.

This is precisely the point at which Life Doctoring becomes so vital and relevant – even if conducted in parallel with medical doctoring. For only Life Doctoring can ensure a true 'healing process' is set into train. Here the role of the Life Doctor is to serve as *midwife* for the patient – helping them to give birth to changes in their sense of self or body identity and not just their body, and to changes in their life as a whole and not just their bodily life.

Life Doctoring sessions serve to support this healing and birthing process by offering times and ways for the patient to step back from purely biomedical diagnoses, prognoses and treatments of their illness and by helping them both feel into and come to understand the deeper meaning and purpose of their illness – thus restoring the health process in place of the illness process. The Life Doctor can also play a vital role in helping the patient to consider more carefully and if necessary reject potentially dangerous or high-risk forms of diagnostic testing, treatment or surgery. For the danger is that these may either miscarry, worsen the patient's symptoms or hasten the progression of their disease – and in any one of these ways result in their premature death. On the other hand, even if medical treatments for serious or terminal diseases *are* 'successful' in purely biomedical terms, they may massively reduce the patient's *quality of life* – merely to extend that life for what is often only a very minimal period.

The Focus of Life Medicine –
The Lived Body

"It is the great error of Western philosophers that they always regard the human body intellectually, from the outside, as though it were not indissolubly a part of the active self."
Sato Tsuji

Which body is it with which we feel ourselves – our self?

Which body is it through which we feel ourselves inwardly 'closer' or more 'distant' to others, however near or far they are in physical space and time?

Which body is it with which we can feel ourselves to be inwardly 'warmer' or 'cooler' towards other people, irrespective of our physical temperature?

Which body is it with which we can feel ourselves inwardly as 'heavier' or 'lighter', 'fatter' or 'thinner', yet without any change to our physical weight or size?

Which body is it whose 'heart' can be inwardly felt as 'big' or 'small', 'warm' or 'cold', with which we or others can feel 'heartened' or 'disheartened', 'lose heart' or suffer 'heartache', seem 'heartless' or 'big hearted' – independently of the size or functioning of 'the heart' as a physical organ?

Which body is it with which we can feel ourselves 'expanding' or 'shrinking', 'uplifted' or 'carried away', 'sucked in' or 'trapped', 'open' or 'closed off', 'full' or 'empty', 'shapeless' or 'spineless', 'exploding' or 'imploding' – yet without our physical body moving or changing shape in any way?

Which body is it with which we can feel inwardly 'drawn into', 'drawn out of' – or 'withdrawn into' ourselves – as if into some warm and nurturing womb or else some cold and solitary prison or tomb?

Which body is it with which we feel 'high' or 'low', 'up' or 'down', 'uplifted' or 'let down', 'beside ourselves', 'spaced out' or confined in our skins?

Which body is it whose 'skin' we feel more or less inwardly 'at home' in, which can make someone seem 'thick- or thin-skinned', that without any physical skin irritations can make us feel 'prickly', 'edgy' or 'irritable', 'stretched' or 'frayed', that can feel tight and constricting like a diving suit or straightjacket – or like a porous, comfortable and loose-fitting garment?

Which body is it that can be felt as more or less inwardly 'solid' or 'firm', 'fluid' or 'airy', 'hard' or 'soft', 'smooth' and 'rounded' or 'jagged' and 'sharp edged' – all independently of its physical shape and features?

Which body is it with which we feel the inner 'brightness' or 'darkness', 'levity' or 'gravity', 'lightness' or 'heaviness' of our own and other peoples' moods?

Which body is it whose overall mood or 'feeling tone' – like its voice tone – can be felt as 'bright or dark', 'light or heavy', 'sharp' or 'dull' and 'flat', 'resonant' and 'full' or 'hollow' and 'empty'?

Which body is it that we actually sense and feel from within, that is the source of all bodily self-perception or 'proprioception' – rather than a mere external object of perception?

The answer to all these questions is not our fleshly 'physical' body and its organs. It is not any body we can measure, weigh or apply any form of medical tests to.

Nor, however, is it some form of pseudo-physical 'energy body' of the sort that New Agers and practitioners of alternative medicine speak of (see *'Life Medicine and 'Energy Medicine'*).

Instead it is our 'felt body' or 'lived body '. To be more exact, it is not just a body we feel or are aware of. Instead it is a body *of* awareness – of feeling awareness or 'soul'.

What I call *feeling awareness* is what used to be called 'soul' or 'psyche' – yet in a way that traditionally has failed to recognise the 'soul' or 'psyche' *as* a body in its own right – the 'lived body' that can also be called our 'soul body' or 'psychic body'.

This body is not composed of tissue, bone and blood, cells and organs. Nor is it made up of some form of 'etheric' or 'subtle' matter. The 'stuff' of which it is made is the 'stuff' that Shakespeare spoke of – that "stuff on which dreams are made" – awareness.

The lived body is therefore also the body as we experience it in our dreams – what Arnold Mindell calls the 'dreambody' or 'dreaming body'.

It is also the very 'life and soul' of our so-called physical body – being also *its* soul or consciousness.

A *portion* of our 'lived body' or 'psychic body' makes up what can be called the 'physical soul' or 'body consciousness ', i.e. those patterns and qualities of molecular and cellular *awareness* that constitute the essence of the human organism.

As for the so-called 'physical body' this is just the lived body and its physical soul as perceived "from the outside".

It is the lived body or psychic body that quite literally 'informs' the physical soul. And yet the lived body *as a whole* is not in any way bounded by it, but is a much *larger* body of feeling awareness, one whose *field* of awareness that embraces our entire life world – including not just our own body but every other body within it – whether than of a person, animal, tree or any *seemingly* insentient object.

Our body consciousness or physical soul too, is in no way unaware of our external environment. Instead it is highly conscious of and sensitive to it – indeed more conscious of it than most people's 'conscious minds' are.

The 'lived body' or 'felt body' should not be thought of simply as referring to the 'physical body' as we feel or experience it from within.

Instead it is the other way round. For again, what we call the 'physical body' is nothing but one dimension and one *portion* of the lived body as it appears to us and others "from the outside" – in the external form of the human body and its organs.

No amount of precise chemical or electromagnetic analysis of the ink marks on the pages of a book or the text on a computer screen will ever reveal the totally invisible, immeasurable and multi-dimensional world of meaning they express.

Similarly, no form of 'objective' external or even 'internal' examination or scanning of the physical body and its organs – which means viewing the inside of the physical body "from the outside" – will ever reveal the lived body – which is a distinct *subjective body* in its own right.

So to persuade a 'scientific' biologist that behind what appears "from the outside" as a mere 3-dimensional physical body lies an invisible body of *living* and *feeling awareness* is like trying to persuade *someone who has not learned to read* that behind the 3-dimensional 'body' of a book or a 2-dimensional screen of text lies an invisible, unbounded and multidimensional world of *living and felt meaning*.

Just as the physical body can be compared to a book or text, so is it also a *speech organ* of the soul and of its body – the lived body or 'soul body' and that portion of it that makes up our 'physical soul'.

Body language or 'body speech', bodily metaphors and physical symptoms are all ways in which the human 'physical' body or organism reveals itself as a living *bio-logical* expression of the lived body and of that portion of it which constitutes our 'physical soul' or 'body consciousness' – being quite literally its 'life speech' or *bios logos* - what Freud called 'organ speech' (*Organsprache*).

This truth finds expression in language itself - for example in bodily metaphor s such as 'losing heart' or finding something 'hard to 'stomach'. These verbal metaphors which are actually not 'metaphors' at all but express directly experienced states of the *lived body*.

These states *also* find symbolic expression in the illness – as for example 'loss of heart' can find expression in heart disease or finding something 'difficult to stomach' in digestive problems. Recognising this is the basis of Life Medicine and Life Doctoring.

Disease as 'Organ Speech'

"Through the long succession of millennia, man has not known himself physiologically; he does not know himself even today."

Friedrich Nietzsche

Do failing organs or disturbances to the functioning of their physiological capacities lead to illness – or are organic or physiological functions and capacities the embodiment of capacities of another sort – capacities of feeling awareness?

Thus when we speak of someone 'losing heart', feeling 'disheartened' or 'heart-broken', for example, we are not just using the language of a biological 'organ' – in this case the heart – as a mere metaphor for a psychological state or sense of 'dis-ease '. It is the other way round. Heart disease is itself *a living biological metaphor* of subjective states of dis-ease and distress such as feeling 'heart-broken', 'heartless' or 'cold-hearted'.

Similarly, respiratory disorders such as asthma arise from a subjective sense of feeling 'stifled' or 'having no room to breathe' in our lives, just as digestive disorders are the expression of aspects of our lived experience and life world that we do not feel able to 'stomach' or 'digest' in our awareness.

Biological medicine seeks 'organic' causes for illness in dysfunctions of our *physiological organs* – and sees even psychological disorders as the result of such organic dysfunctions, as disorders of our brain chemistry. As a result, biological medicine is blind to the deeper meaning and truth of the bodily language and 'metaphors' we use to describe what are usually thought of only as 'mental' or 'psychological' feelings and states. It does not see that the language of these bodily metaphors is a way of recognising that the physical body and its organs are not a biological machine or a mere product of our genes but a *living biological language* of the human being.

In contrast, Freud spoke of bodily symptoms as a type of organic *language* or 'organ speech' (*Organsprache*). Similarly, Life Medicine recognises all organs and functions of the 'physical' body as the biological expression of organised capacities and functions of another body – our 'lived body' – the body of our feeling awareness of all that we experience in our lives.

In German there are not one but two words for 'the body' – *Körper* and *Leib*. The only equivalents of *Körper* in English are the words 'corpus' and 'corpse'. 'Corpse' is also the root meaning of the Greek word 'soma', from which the term 'somatic' derives. It refers of course to a dead body as opposed to a living one. There is however another German word for body – *Leib* – that can be translated as 'lived body' or 'life' body – for it is part of a whole family of words to do with 'life' (*Leben*) and 'living' (*leben*). These words include *erleben* ('to experience') and *Erlebnis* (an experience). Through the inner lens of the German language in other words, life (*Leben*) and living (*leben*) are understood essentially as realm of *subjective experiencing* (*er-leben*). Thus the body as *Leib* or 'lived body' refers to our own 'experienced' and 'experiencing' body' – the body of our living *experience* of ourselves, our lives and our entire life world. The basic 'capacities' of the lived body or *Leib* therefore have to do with what we are or are not able to do with our experience (*Erlebnis*) of living (*leben*), of life (*Leben*) and of our 'life world' (*Lebenswelt*).

In physiological terms, the capacities of the lived body are our capacity to *sense, perceive, breathe in, digest* and *metabolise* all that we experience, allowing it to *circulate* within our awareness and thus *nourish* our very *being* with life-giving *meaning*.

146

Both our sense organs and other biological organs such as our lungs, stomach and heart, together with their corresponding physiological functions, are essentially nothing but organic and physiological *embodiments* of capacities belonging to our lived body as a 'psychical organism' or 'body of awareness' – an awareness *more or less* open to or capable of sensuously embracing, feeling and perceiving, breathing in, digesting and metabolising all that we experience in our lives – and in this way extracting meaning from it.

On the other hand, any *lack or dysfunction* of these basic capacities of awareness belonging to the lived body may also *embody* itself – finding expression in what biomedicine then sees only as purely 'physiological' or 'organic' dysfunctions, disorders or 'diseases' – for example respiratory, digestive, metabolic or circulatory diseases.

"We cannot say that the organ has capacities, but must say that the capacity has organs... capability, articulating itself into capacities creating organs characterises the organism as such."
Martin Heidegger

The idea that biological organs are a "creation" or embodiment of the very capabilities or capacities we associate with that organ is of course a radical one.

Yet along with the family of German words that includes the 'lived body' (*Leib*), 'life' (*Leben*) and experiencing (*er-leben*) goes another word that hints at how this idea may be understood: the verb 'to body' (*leiben*).

For as Heidegger remarked in addressing a circle of doctors:

"We know by now a great deal – almost more than we can encompass – about what we call the body, without having seriously thought about what <u>bodying</u> is ... The bodying of life is nothing separate by itself, encapsulated in the 'physical mass' in which the body can appear to us..."

Hence also the profound significance of another insight of his, namely that: *"Every feeling is an embodiment attuned in this or that way, a mood that embodies in this or that way."*

It is through the lived body that we quite literally embody or 'body' felt tones or 'moods' of feeling awareness or 'feeling tones' – allowing them to find expression in cellular tone, skin tone, muscle and organ tone, i.e. in 'organ speech' – as well as in the tones of our vocal speech. The lived body then, is the very source and essence of the human 'organism '.

For it is that musical or tonal 'instrument' (the root meaning of the Greek word *organon* from which the term 'organism' is derived) through which we inwardly 'speak' or 'utter' our organs themselves from out of shaped and patterned tones of feeling awareness or 'feeling tones'. For, what are sound, music and speech except a shaping or patterning of tone?

Yet feeling tones can be either healthy and 'sound' or else more or less muddied, discordant and 'unsound'. This is also the reason we speak of someone's health or a particular organ being or not being in 'sound' condition, and associate health with 'soundness', the words *sound* and *soundness* being the root meaning of the German words for 'healthy' and 'health' – ge*sund* and Ge*sund*heit.

The human organism then – indeed *any* organism – is nothing 'biological' or 'organic' in the narrow scientific sense. It is 'biological' only in the essential sense of being that instrument or *organon* through which 'life' (*bios*) speaks itself in the form of fleshly organs – giving physical shape and tone to felt patterns, shapes, tones and textures of feeling awareness.

The essence of any organism consists of *organising field patterns of awareness*. These in turn are what give ordered and organised shape and form to that larger *patterned field of awareness* that constitutes the perceived 'environment' or *life world* of any organism.

Human *language* too is an organised and organising structure, one which shapes and patterns our specifically human awareness and perception of the world. And language itself is made up of 'organising patterns of awareness' that make it an integral part of the lived body – and not a mere function of something we call 'the mind' or of the brain as a biological organ.

It is because it is an integral part of the human organism that the body and its organs itself figure so strongly in *language itself* – in countless everyday expressions relating to bodily *organs* such as the heart (feeling 'disheartened' or 'a stab in the heart), to *parts* of the body ('having one's feet on the ground') and bodily functions such as respiration (feeling 'stifled' or having 'no room to breathe').

The body even figures in the mere use of *simple prepositions* such as 'in' and 'out', 'on' and 'off', 'up' and 'down' – for example being 'onto' or 'into' something', feeling 'up' or 'down', 'high' and 'low', 'off colour' or 'out of' one's mind. For all these expressions arise from and reflect our felt bodily relation to space – as also does the use of words such as 'upset', 'unstable' or 'imbalanced' and expressions such as 'leaning to one side', 'finding one's ground' or 'shifting' one's stance or attitude, posture or position.

This all-pervasive bodily dimension of language itself – and its roots in bodily experiencing – was first explored in depth by Lakoff and Johnson in their book *Metaphors We Live By*. Yet it also lends support to the basic principles of Life Medicine, as well as to Freud 's notion of 'organ speech '. This notion is in turn closely associated with what, in his last years, he came to call 'The Second Fundamental Principle of Psychoanalysis '.

This is the principle that 'bodily' states and symptoms were not merely things that emerged 'parallel' with or 'concomitant' to unconscious mental or 'psychic' states. Instead what were previously thought of in psychoanalysis only as "somatic concomitants" of these states were recognised as "the truly psychical" (Freud).

The radical implication of this principle is that the true foundation and focus of psychoanalysis is not 'the interpretation of dreams' or some mysterious entity called 'the unconscious' but *the language of the body* – which finds expression both in our waking life and in our dreams and 'dreaming body' and is the symbolic key to all forms and symptoms of illness.

Yet the significance of Freud's new 'foundational principle of psychoanalysis' has still not been registered by most psychoanalysts or schools of psychoanalysis – and certainly not in medical theory and practice.

Only through the work of the Argentinean psychoanalyst *Luis Chiozza* did psychoanalysis come to both appreciate and apply this principle.

He did so by recognising, as Life Medicine does, that the two *distinct but inseparable* dimensions of what Freud called 'organ speech' – verbal expression such as 'feeling stifled' or 'stabbed in the heart' on the one hand, and experienced physical sensations or symptoms such as breathing difficulties or heart pains on the other – share a *common source*. In other words, symptoms of illness itself are not only reflected in language that describes felt states of dis-ease. Instead illness itself *is* a language.

As a psychoanalyst, Chiozza saw the common source of illness and language as 'the unconscious'. In Life Medicine this common source is seen as life itself – as experienced through the lived body.

Yet it was Chiozza who also first developed a methodological approach to illness akin to Life Doctoring. Derived from Victor von Weizsäcker and called the 'pathobiographical' method, it involves seeking the 'hidden story' behind a patient's illness by finding links between its biology on the one hand, and the biography or life story of the patient on the other. Such links can above all be sought and found through the *language of illness* and through understanding illness itself *as a language*.

References:

Chiozza, Luis A. *Hidden Affects in Somatic Disorders*
Chiozza, Luis A. *Why Do We Fall Ill? – The Story Hiding in the Body*
Heidegger, Martin, *Zollikon Seminars*
Lakoff and Johnson, *Metaphors We Live By*

The Language of Illness

Could it be that the way we use language to talk *about* illness and disease affects our whole understanding of it? Could it be that "the essence of a disease" and "the essence of a word" – of the language with which we describe states of 'dis-ease' – are one and the same?

To begin with it is important to recognise how many phrases used to talk about illness contain words that imply that it is:

- some 'thing' that we 'have', 'catch' or 'get'
- something that is 'wrong' or 'bad'
- something that attacks us
- Something that fails

Examples:

- I *caught* a cold.
- She *has* cancer.
- What's *wrong* with me?
- He's got a *bad* heart.
- My back/head is *killing* me.
- He is suffering from liver *failure.*

Secondly, biological medicine, far from being based purely on scientific fact, is pervaded by verbal metaphors or figures of speech – and in particular expressions derived from the language of *war*.

Examples:

- *War* on cancer.
- *Defending or protecting oneself against* disease.
- *Battling, struggling or fighting against* an illness.
- *Mobilising/reinforcing* the body's immune *defences.*
- An *aggressive* tumour or virus.
- *Fighting off* an infection.
- *Killer* cells.

Thirdly, illness has been explained and interpreted historically in many different religious, moral and 'scientific' ways.

Examples:

- As a punishment for sin.
- As a 'test' of will or faith.
- As an attack by malign spirits.
- As a result of misdeeds in a past life.
- As a sign of moral 'degeneracy' (syphilis, AIDS).
- As an evolutionary means for the survival of the fittest.
- As an invasion by pathogens such as bacteria or viruses.
- As the 'price' paid for an 'unhealthy' lifestyle.
- As a result of eating the 'wrong' foods.
- As a colonisation by cancerous cells.
- As a result of faulty genes.

Fourthly, the body itself has been culturally and linguistically described in many different ways:

Examples:

- As an image of God.
- As a sacred temple of the gods.
- As something to be controlled or tamed by the mind.
- As a container of emotions and of the soul or psyche.
- As a mere disposable shell of the soul or spirit.
- As a more or less well-functioning machine.
- As a product of our genes.

Body Language in Everyday Speech

Everyday speech and verbal language is itself full of 'body language' – containing countless metaphors or 'figures of speech' which not only refer to bodily organs and functions but offer symbolic clues to types of inner dis-ease that might find expression in both physical and mental health problems.

Examples:

- To be/feel *inflamed*, to be *thick-skinned* or *thin-skinned*, *sensitive* or *prickly*, *irritable* or *itchy*, to be *touched* or *untouched* by something/someone, to let something/someone *get under one's skin*.

- To be *heartless* or *cold-hearted*, to *take something to heart*, to be *disheartened*, to *lack heart* or *lose heart*, to be *heartbroken*, a *heartfelt* emotion, a *fluttering heart* etc.

- To find something hard to *stomach* or *digest*, to feel *sick* or *nauseated* about something, to have a *gut feeling* about something, to feel *gutted*.

- To not feel one can *breathe freely*, to feel *stifled*, to feel one has *no room to breathe*, to lack *breathing space*, to lack *inspiration* (from the Latin *spirare* – to breathe).

- To be *headstrong*, to be *boneheaded*, to keep *a clear head*, to *head* in a certain direction, to make or not to make *headway*, to *head something off*, to *have a head* for something, to *lose one's head*, to *bring something to a head* etc.

- To be unable to *face* or *face up* to something or someone, to come *face to face* with something or someone, to *show one's true face*.

- To not *see* a point, to refuse to *see* something, to not *see straight*, to not *see* things in perspective, to lack *vision* or *insight*, to be *short-sighted*, to *close one's eyes* to something, to have a *blindspot*, to not have an *eye* for something.

- To stand on one's own *two feet*, to find one's *balance* or *ground*, to *stand up* for oneself, to take things *in one's stride*.

- To lack *backbone,* to be *spineless,* to *back* someone up or to be in need of support and *backing.*

- To feel inwardly *frozen stiff* or *immobilised.*

- To *shoulder* a burden or lean on someone's shoulders.

- To feel something as a *pain in the neck* or a *pain in the ass.*

- To feel *overstretched, stressed, stiff, constricted* or *tense.*

- To feel someone *getting up one's nose.*

- To be unable to *handle* or *get a grip* on a situation or person.

- To be full of bile.

Even simple linguistic prepositions such as 'in' and 'out', 'on' and 'off', 'up' and 'down' etc – all of which form part and parcel of the very structure of language – play a particularly significant role here, implying that the body is a container of some sort for mental and emotional objects.

Examples:

letting something 'out', taking or holding something 'in', having an idea 'in' one's mind or a feeling 'in' one's body, letting 'out' an emotion, feeling 'off' or 'put off', going 'into' oneself or letting things 'out of' oneself, feeling 'up' or 'down', 'high' or 'low', trapped 'in' one's body or 'out of' one's mind.

All these expressions arise from and reflect our felt bodily relation to space – as also does the use of words such as *'upset', 'unstable'* or *'imbalanced'* and expressions such as *'leaning to one side', 'finding one's ground'* or *'shifting'* one's stance, attitude, posture or position.

That language itself *is* 'body language' can also be seen from the way in which expressions referring to 'mental' states make use of figures of speech but relating to specific bodily sensations or movements:

Examples:

feeling 'overstretched' or 'under pressure', 'reaching' for a goal, 'catching' or 'catching onto' something, 'running away' from something', 'moving on' and 'getting ahead', 'falling behind' or 'going downhill', 'falling apart' or putting oneself 'together', 'shaking' with fear or 'shaking' something off, 'shifting' one's attitude, 'carrying' a heavy burden, 'grasping', 'hanging onto', 'losing one's grip on' or 'letting go' of something etc.

These are examples of a whole range of expressions used to refer to 'mental' states which at the same time refer to *muscular* states. For example we speak of feeling *tense* or *relaxed*, or else *nervous* or *restless* – hence wanting to fidget or make use of our muscles in some way.

Similarly, a state of high tension or anxiety may be felt muscularly – for example as a 'tension headache ', a 'knot' in the stomach, a 'flutter' in the heart etc. This is not surprising given that our heart, stomach and intestines are made up of *muscle* – as are our respiratory and vocal organs.

If someone is drunk or drugged is it their mind or their muscles that may make them feel disoriented or lose their balance? Perhaps it is both and neither. Perhaps it is a person's overall or underlying bodily mood or *tone of feeling* which finds expression both in *muscle tone* and in *mental states.*

Hence also the expression 'highly strung' – which can apply to both a person's nerves and their muscles, but is drawn from the language of stringed musical instruments – and suggests an understanding of the human body or 'organism' itself as a musical instrument – the meaning of the Greek word *organon.*

Finally, both our language and our muscles and joints can be more or less rigid and stiff or *articulate* – allowing us to freely communicate or 'articulate' ourselves through both verbal speech, different tones of voice and 'body speech '. Could it be then, that both illness and language, bodily symptoms and bodily figures of speech – what Foucault called "the essence of a disease" and the "essence of a word" – are one and the same? Could it be that illness gives this common essence the form of symptoms, whilst language gives it the form of bodily metaphors or figures of speech? Could it be that the body itself is a not a biological machine to be repaired but a *living language* of the human being? For verbal language, as we have seen, is itself largely 'body language' – being made up of figures of speech rooted in bodily sensations and states.

Illness as a Language and 'Somatic Metaphor' – Cases from the work of Dr. Brian Broom

The following case reports are drawn from Dr. Brian Broom's book *Meaning-full Disease – how personal experience and meanings can cause and maintain physical illness.* They are based on the approach to illness taught by Brian Broom to health professionals at the Auckland University of Technology and first detailed in his book *Somatic Illness – the Patient's Other Story* – which contains a wealth of further case descriptions. Broom's 'MindBody' approach – like that of Life Doctoring – consists in exploring the nature of a patient's illness as 'somatic metaphor'. This means listening for and hearing in the patient's *own language and choice of words* evidence of clear metaphorical connections between the patient's somatic symptoms on the one hand and particular events and experiences in their lives on the other. In all the cases that follow, names of patients have been changed and any similarity to persons known to you reflects the commonness of such connections but also the essentially symbolic nature of illness as 'somatic metaphor'.

Skin thickening

Eunice, a 71 year old woman, had an 18 month history of generalized thickening of the skin, and tissues under the skin, causing uncomfortable splinting of the chest, and tightness of the arms and upper legs. This thickening was very obvious. Despite her age it was impossible to pinch her skin into folds. Despite intensive investigation a firm diagnosis had not been made. I will not emphasise the medical detail but though the appearances were not classical she was told she had "connective tissue disease" and was accordingly treated with steroids and other potent drugs.

I was asked to see her for a second opinion. I began by enquiring about the onset of her skin thickening. She startled me by saying that it began when she fell over in the local garden nursery, sustaining injuries to her face and legs. I was inclined to brush this information off, and get on with the important (sic) material. But something made me hesitate, and I enquired further. She described the fall as "shattering." Mystified as to the relevance of this I asked what effect this event had had on her. She replied: " I went into my shell for a while." I was immediately struck by the fact she was presenting to me with a thickened shell of skin and here she was using language to match. I invited further comment, and within the next 3 to 4 minutes she used the words "I went into my shell" 3 times. Moreover, she further volunteered in her description of being taken back to her home by a friendly gentleman: "I went inside the four walls of my house, and closed the door, and sat and sat and sat." In the few weeks following the injury skin thickening developed first in the legs and then became more generalized. I sat listening to this wondering what sense to make of it. I enquired about aspects of her life. She had enjoyed very good health throughout her life, but it seems that the accident compromised ("shattered") her sense of herself as perennially invulnerable. Moreover the embarrassing injuries to her face induced social withdrawal. She had actually started to improve by the time I saw her and the possibility existed that this was a response to the drugs she had been on. I enquired of her as to what she felt was the cause of her improvement. She related it to a friend who had come to her and said that she should get active again. She said that she improved again as she started to "come out of my shell." This "shell" theme was the metaphor she persisted with in both her language and her body.

I suggested to her that the thickening of the skin was a bodily (somatic) representation of what she was also expressing in using the term "shell." She accepted this, though without much insight. I encouraged her to continue to be active and resume her previous social contacts, and suggested I follow her up regularly for support, encouragement, explanation, education, and revision of her home situation so that coping could be ensured for as long as possible. After the third visit she declined further sessions. One year later both she and her physician reported marked clinical improvement, and she was on no medication.

Leukoplakia

Teresa requests review because she wants to 'live life more fully'. In her thirties she developed leukoplakia, a precancerous condition of the mouth. By the time she came to me she had had seven surgical interventions, including removal of carcinoma and one plastic reconstructions of the tongue and the floor of the mouth--the last requiring eighteen months rehabilitation as she learned to speak again. Early in the interview she proffered the interesting comment that "if only I could get rid of it (my emphasis) I would be able to live more fully from day to day". Though she was obviously (!) referring to the leukoplakia and cancerous tendency I suspected the it was not the cancer that had been removed 2 years before, with no evidence of recurrence. I noted the words but made no comment.

A review of her life-story was illuminating, and some key points will be emphasised. Apparently, after she was born, she and her mother were collected by father from the hospital. He dropped them off at home and went off to see his mistress. When Teresa was seven years old her father suicided, though she was not aware of the nature of his death. At age twelve she was crying in her bedroom. Mother found her, asked what was wrong, and Teresa replied that she was crying about "daddy". Mother, who was now alcoholic, responded: "It's your fault your father is dead – you would never sit on his knee." The background to this cruel comment is not clear. Teresa did remember that as a child she often felt much more identified with her absent father than with her mother. At age sixteen she learned from relatives that her father died by suicide. At nineteen she entered a marriage that, over six years, repeated in some ways the traumas of childhood. At age thirty three she developed the leukoplakia of the mouth. It turns out that this was the age that her father committed suicide. Her father was an oral surgeon. I point this out to Teresa who has herself wondered, over the years, whether this is significant, though it had never been discussed with doctors. Returning in my mind to the **it** referred to above, I asked her what, apart from this cancerous tendency, she would most like to get rid of in her life. She seemed to understand what I was asking, but struggled initially, becoming very tearful, unable to find the right word. Eventually she said she most wanted to get rid of *the shame.* To me it seemed likely that the shame and the leukoplakia were intimately connected in some way. Could one think up a better somatic metaphor than a precancerous condition of the mouth, for the shame of being responsible for the death of one's oral surgeon father?

Teresa had some brief psychotherapy, which was unusually fast-moving and involved only nine sessions. The turning point in therapy occurred when she actually started to remember sitting on her father's knee. She reported, after the session in which that occurred, a persistent "joy" which has continued, and seems to have expressed itself in a variety of interpersonal and social freedoms. A year later she reported no further problems and her surgeon expressed astonishment with the good state of her mouth.

Nasal irritation

Katrina, a woman in her twenties has struggled with obesity since age thirteen. Finally she conquers it by having a gastric bypass operation, losing some 60 kilograms in weight. At last the obesity is behind her. But the problems associated with her obesity appear in another form. She works as an acupuncturist. Since losing weight, and transcending her enormous weight problem, she has become more and more irritable with clients who seek her help for what she sees as relatively trivial bodily concerns. Compared to her struggle with obesity many of these clients have little to complain about. She no longer wants to tussle with 'bodies'. As this irritability increases she develops chronic nose and sinus catarrh, congestion, and infections resistant to antibiotics. She *can hardly bear to face* some of these clients. Her nose may settle for a while when away from clients, but as soon as she leans over these troublesome clients demanding solutions to their 'trivial' problems her nose starts to pour fluid. They get *up my nose*.

Vertebral arthritis

A couple were referred because of marital difficulty ... In the course of the first session he complained of back-pain, and we enquired further about this. He had been previously diagnosed with ankylosing spondylitis, which is an inflammatory arthritis of the vertebral column leading, eventually, to a rigid fusion of all the vertebrae. Asked when the problem began, without any hesitation he gave the following intriguing story. Seven years before he had been present at his wife's first labour, during which an epidural anesthetic was given. He was absolutely appalled at the sight of the needle being inserted into his wife's spinal column, and collapsed in a faint on to the floor. He woke up with pain in his back, and had been "feeling her pain" ever since.

Getting to the Heart of Illness –
and of Heart Disease

Listed on the next page is an extended set of everyday expressions, many of which are mentioned in other sections of this book and all of which refer to the 'heart'. Together they 'get to the heart' of what I call the 'felt body' or 'lived body '. For the 'heart' they refer to is not a mere biological organ which mechanically pumps blood, and neither do the expressions refer merely to 'states of mind' separate from and independent of the body. Instead the 'heart' they all refer to is an organ of our lived body rather than our 'physical body'. It is the heart experienced not as a biological organ but as the 'heart' of the lived body – understood as *an organ of feeling awareness.*

"The Language of the Heart"

'a loving heart'

'a passionate heart'

a 'big heart' / a 'kind heart'

a 'cold heart' / 'cold-hearted'

a 'warm heart' / 'warm-hearted'

to be 'open hearted' or 'closed-hearted'

to be 'heart-broken' or 'broken-hearted'

to 'go to' or 'get to' the heart of something'

to be 'hard-hearted' or to 'harden one's heart'

to have or not have the 'heart' for something

to suffer an 'aching heart' or 'heartache'

to be 'heartened' or 'disheartened'

to 'lose heart' or to 'lack heart'

to have a 'heart-to-heart' talk

to feel 'stabbed in the heart'

to 'take something to heart'

to 'strengthen one's heart'

to speak 'from the heart'

to feel one's heart 'sink'

a 'heartfelt emotion'

to be 'heartless'

a 'frozen heart'

'At the heart' of Life Medicine lie three basic understandings all linking Language, Life and Illness:

1. That everyday language referring to *any* of the parts, organs or functions of the human body does not merely make use of bodily 'metaphor s' to describe mental or emotional states, but instead indicates the way we live and experience such states in a bodily way – through our subjectively felt body or 'lived body'.
2. That *both* bodily expressions such as 'losing heart' *and* bodily conditions such as heart disease and its symptoms are *symbols* of something else – states and experiences of the felt or lived body and of *its* organs and functions.
3. That so-called 'organic' dysfunctions, disorders or diseases – for example heart diseases – are biological embodiments of basic dysfunctions, disorders or diseases of the lived or felt body: for example an incapacity to feel or love expressed through a hardened heart, or the felt experience of a 'broken heart' or 'loss of heart'.

Life Medicine therefore, does *not* claim that illness is 'all in the mind'. On the contrary, it understands illness – like the many everyday expressions that symbolise its nature and symptoms – as an expression of our subjective experience of life and of our subjectively felt body – 'the lived body'.

No form of conventional medical *testing* however, no matter how technologically sophisticated, can see, scan or diagnose the felt or lived body – nor can it detect a felt sense of *dis-ease* in *that* body – such as a 'broken heart' or a feeling of 'loss of heart'.

Similarly, no form of biomedical *treatment* for hardened arteries can cure 'a hardened heart', just as no form of 'open-heart' surgery can cure someone with 'a closed heart'.

"The heart is often described as a type of pump. With the latest developments in modern technology, there are all kinds of heart operations that can be performed, even the use of heart transplants. In many cases, even when hearts are repaired through medical technology, the same trouble reoccurs at a later date, or the patient recovers only to fall prey to a different, nearly fatal or fatal disease. This is not always the case by any means, but when such a person does recover fully, and maintains good health, it is because [their] beliefs, attitudes and feelings have changed for the better, and because the person 'has a heart' again; in other words because the patient himself has regained the will to live."

"Many people who have heart trouble feel that they have 'lost the heart' for life. They may feel broken-hearted for many reasons. They may feel heartless, or imagine themselves to be so cold-hearted that they punish themselves literally by trying to lose their heart."

"With many people having such difficulties, the addition of love in the environment may work far better than any heart operation. A new pet given to a bereaved individual has saved more people from needing heart operations than any physician. In other words, a 'love transplant' in the environment may work far better overall than a heart-transplant operation, or a bypass, or whatever; in such ways the heart is allowed to heal itself."

"The condition of your heart is affected, for example, by your own feelings about it. If you consider yourself to be cold-hearted or heartless, those feelings will have a significant effect upon that physical organ. If you feel broken-hearted then you will also have that feeling reflected in one way or another in the physical organ itself.... each individual also has many options open. Everyone who feels broken-hearted does not necessarily die of heart failure for example. The subject of health cannot be considered in an isolated fashion ... each person will try to fulfil their own unique abilities, and to 'fill out' the experience of life as fully as possible."

from *The Way Toward Health* by Jane Roberts (see appendix 6)

Case Example 3

A recently bereaved widow, whose husband Harry died from a heart attack, finds herself suffering disturbing chest pains at night and goes to see her physician. The physician sees her symptoms only as signs of some possible organic disorder which might be 'causing' them. He sends her to a consultant to test for possible heart conditions. The tests proving inconclusive, the consultant ends up diagnosing mild angina, and prescribes beta-blockers. These in turn prove to have little effect on the patient's symptoms.

On visiting her physician a second time however, the latter recalls her recent bereavement and, as a result, begins to read the bodily 'text' of her symptoms in a different way, understanding them in the life context of her loss and the pain it may be causing her. Rather than seeking a purely clinical 'diagnosis' of the patient's symptoms he himself listens to his patient in a genuinely patient way. As a result an insight flashes through his mind which he shares with her. He 'sees' that she may be suffering from a doubly *broken heart*: "the one that killed Harry, and the one you're left alive with, that hurts when you're most alone in the middle of the night...the broken heart that gave up and the one that has to carry on painfully." This *heartfelt* hearing of the patient and the *heart-to-heart* talk that ensue are the first time anyone has ever acknowledged the pain of her grief. It gives her the *strength of heart* to acknowledge and bear it in a new way. Her symptoms disappear. The patient's heart symptoms disappear as bodily symbols and metaphorical signifiers of her pained heart, not through an intellectual understanding of their significance alone but through a memory arising from the *feeling heart* of the physician.

This paradigmatic case vignette, cited by Dr David Zigmond in an article on different modes of patient-physician communication, goes to the heart of the contrast between biomedical diagnosis and what could be called 'life diagnosis'.

The root meaning of the term 'diagnosis' actually is 'through knowledge' (*dia-gnosis*). Yet the Greek verb, *gignostikein,* from which the word *gnosis* (knowledge) derives did not mean merely knowledge of or about something – (for example biomedical knowledge of the body). Instead it denoted the sort of knowing we refer to when we speak of being 'familiar' with people, of 'knowing' them well or intimately as human beings – in much the same way that family doctors used to know or be familiar with their patients, as if a part of their families.

It was this type of 'knowing' that the doctor in Zigmond's case study brought to bear in relating to the widow – not just his standard body of medical knowledge 'about' the heart as a biological organ and the type of 'diagnosis' to which it can lead. His method consisted simply of having the patience to listen to his patient in a different way – not seeking a diagnosis of a possible heart 'condition' but affirming her *heartbreak* in a *heartfelt* way. By 'bearing with' his patient in this way, helping to bear the burden of her pained heart with her – she no longer felt herself so painfully alone in bearing it – and was able to find a *new bearing* towards the bereavement that occasioned it.

The paradox that Zigmond notes however, is that despite the inconclusiveness of the initial medical tests, had the physician himself not embodied this new and different bearing towards his patient – had he not heard her in a *heartfelt* way as a human being but simply treated her as a potential 'case' of angina – then the patient herself might well have found herself in the position of having no way to express the heartbreak of her loss *except* through actual and perhaps increasingly acute cardiac symptoms – using her biological heart as an instrument of what Freud called 'organ speech '.

The physician's capacity for a different type of listening – one that did not merely serve as a prelude to some form of purely biomedical diagnosis was therefore 'preventative medicine' in the deepest sense. For it may well have forestalled a process whereby this patient might well have ended up as a genuine 'heart case' requiring serious medical intervention. Alternatively, she might have found herself seen as a so-called 'heart sink' patient – someone who repeatedly 'bothers' her doctor, but whose medical tests continue to reveal no conclusive, measurable signs of any organic disorder or heart disease – thus suggesting some form of malingering. Yet such 'heart-sink' patients are not a marginal group. In their persistence, they are simply unconsciously reacting to the absence of a type of listening that most patients actually seek – the type of listening required for 'life diagnosis' and 'life doctoring'.

This one single case described by Zigmond is therefore 'paradigmatic' – for in its simplicity it nevertheless reveals in full clarity the sharply opposing frameworks or 'paradigms' of Biological Medicine and Life Medicine, Bio-medical Doctoring and Life Doctoring. Indeed recent research has shown that many older widows die within three years of their bereavement – not due to arterial disease but principally through an enlargement of the heart's pumping chamber – in other words a (painfully) 'throbbing heart'.

Zigmond also offers us a study in the very meaning of 'diagnosis' as such – showing how different ways of listening to and coming to 'know' a patient can themselves have a direct bearing on the patient's health and medical condition itself. Our *biology* has its basis in our *biography*, and in that larger *body of awareness* that is our *life world* as a whole. For it is always within the specific contexts of our life world that we experience a felt 'dis-ease ', just as it is *capacities of awareness* that allow us to relate to and respond to our life world in a healthy way – *with* awareness.

Illness can and has been understood in many ways: in a purely objective and biomedical way, as a mechanical, neurophysiological 'effect' of psychical stress or trauma, as a relation to our life world and other people in it, as a form of silent bodily *communication* or even protest, as blocked action or communication, and/or as a metaphorical *language* through which we give silent bodily *expression* to any *subjectively* felt 'dis-ease '. Understanding organic illness as a language of awareness embraces all other understandings of it. More importantly it provides us with an understanding of illness that affirms its innate *meaningfulness* in the life of the individual – as an expression and embodiment of their lived experience of themselves and of their life world as a whole, as an expression and embodiment of the degree of awareness they bring to their experience, and as an expression and embodiment too, of the specific capacities or 'organs' of awareness that they do or do not exercise in relating and responding to their experienced self and world – for it is these specific capacities that offer new keys to diagnosing illness *as* a language. (see The Language of Illness and Illness as a Language)

Reference:

Dr David Zigmond *Three Types of Encounter in the Healing Arts: Dialogue, Dialectic and Didacticism*

Life Medicine and Organic Impairment

It is the organising or 'ordering' capacities of the lived body and physical soul that allow us not just to remain open to, sense and feel, take and breathe in, digest and metabolise our experience of life but also to:

(a) *make sense* of our lives and life world in an organised and ordered way, and

(b) *engage in* our lives and relate to our life world in a meaningful and fulfilling way. This is achieved through what the existential physician and neurologist Kurt Goldstein called "ordered performances".

By this he meant ordered activities or patterns of action of any sort that we are normally able to enact within or in response to our life world or environment – whether basic actions such as breathing, moving, walking, talking, clothing ourselves, cooking, eating or fulfilling domestic tasks etc., or more sophisticated 'performances' such as engaging in highly skilled creative, communicative or professional activities and interactions.

Chronic or permanent loss of or impairment to organs and organic functions (for example loss of mobility, sight or hearing) impair and limit such ordered life activities or 'performances'. They also affect and express states of our *organism as a whole* and are felt through 'generalised' organismic states such as fatigue, depression, loss of cognitive capacities or libido etc.

From the perspective of Life Medicine however, to see biological 'death' resulting from organ failure as the end point of our being or existence is to forget that the lived body, being a non-physical body of feeling awareness or soul – our 'soul body' – is by nature eternal.

Therefore what is essentially threatened by a continued or worsening organic impairment – even if 'life threatening' – is not any form of 'absolute death' but rather what is of absolute importance to the current *life* and *health* of the patient in this life and this world i.e. their capacity to *actualise their individual potentials* by means of specific organic capacities and the ordered 'performances' or patterns of action they facilitate. For as Goldstein wrote:

"...health is not an objective condition which can be understood by the methods of natural science alone. It is rather a condition related to the mental attitude by which the individual has to value what is essential for his life. 'Health' appears thus as a value; its value consists in the individual's capacity to actualise his nature to the degree, that for him at least, is essential."

If this understanding offers us a deeper insight into the true essence of 'health', what then are its implications for our understanding of the essence of 'illness'? In the context of organic impairment this question takes us beyond the purely clinical realm of biological medicine and takes us once again into the realm of personal *life meaning.*

For example, a partial loss of movement in a leg may *mean* very little to a sedentary worker but *everything* to an athlete such as a runner or sportsman, just as a speech impairment may mean much less to a manual labourer but everything to a salesman, teacher or writer – inducing an overall organismic reaction that Goldstein calls 'catastrophic' shock and anxiety – being a threat to the very essence of the individual's 'life' or 'existence' understood *as a means of self-actualisation*. On the other hand a patient may be known to have a 'disease' in a potentially 'life threatening' cancer *without this in any way* outwardly affecting their capacity for self-actualisation through specific patterns of action or organised 'performances'. If, as a result of this 'disease' diagnosis however, the life world and life possibilities of the cancer

172

patient are shrunk down to merely being kept alive in a hospital bed and/or subject to hi-tech radiological or chemotherapeutic treatments which radically reduce their quality of life – then it is difficult to argue that this type of 'medicine' in any way benefits their 'health' in the sense defined by Goldstein.

As for illness or 'disease', he writes:

"It may be stated as certain that any disease is an abnormality but not that every abnormality is a disease."

So for example, when people get ill through 'stress' i.e. when demands far beyond what Goldstein calls their "average potentialities" are imposed on them – they may recognise an *abnormality* in their condition, for example feel ill with the symptoms of a cold or flu – *an ailment* – but they do not regard themselves for this reason as having 'a disease'.

In general however, whatever 'symptoms' may be observed, such as high blood pressure, or whatever 'diseases' may be bio-medically diagnosed as a result – for example heart disease – all that has actually occurred is a deviation from a *biological norm*.

Yet this scientific norm may have little to do with a patient's own highly *individual* norm for assessing their own 'health' – understood as their capacity to lead a healthy and fulfilling life.

What biomedicine judges by its own purely *biological norms* to be a 'disease' therefore, is in essence nothing more than an observable *change of state* of the organism, one that may not only be more or less temporary – but also more or less meaningful, threatening or catastrophic to a patient's experience of *life* – not just the life of their physical body.

For as Seth explains (see appendix 6)

"The body does not recognise <u>diseases as diseases</u> in usually understood terms. It regards all activity as experience, as a momentary condition of life, as a balancing situation." (from *The Way Toward Health* by Jane Roberts)

Yet biological medicine understands its primary purpose as to fight disease and prevent death at any cost – qualitative and quantitative – to the life of the patient. This implies that disease is merely and invariably an abnormality with no meaning – and that life itself consists merely in just continuing to 'be alive' or 'survive' biologically, rather than *living* in a way that brings a necessary, minimum degree of self-actualisation and fulfilment (the essence of 'health').

That is why, in cases where a patient is left with a remaining deficit or chronic and incurable organic impairment which more or less severely limits their capacity for a particular type of ordered "performance" or life activity, Goldstein 's view was that it was of the utmost importance for the individual to find ways to re-order and if necessary *limit* their life world itself – what he called their "milieu" – not through mere institutionalisation or for the purposes of medical treatment but in a way that:

a) reduces the demands imposed on the individual to respond with "ordered performances " to an extent they are no longer capable of or can cope with

b) nevertheless provides the patient with an ordered environment in which they can still continue to engage in fulfilling forms of ordered activity, old or new.

Though Goldstein dealt with patients suffering from severe neurological damage, this also applies to people with far less severe illnesses or even minor ailments – to which they might respond by taking days off work, staying at home or in bed etc. – all of which are simple ways of temporarily limiting their life world to a less demanding or stressful "milieu" – but one in which they can nevertheless engage in some satisfactory ordered activities or work of some sort.

'Order' is in this way central to Goldstein's view of organic impairment, suggesting a manner in which the physician could serve as a 'life doctor' in the most literal sense – restoring a minimum degree of healthily fulfilling and ordered activity to the patient's *life* and *well-being* rather than seeking only to cure or alleviate a physical disease or impairment.

"...being well means to be capable of ordered behaviour which may prevail in spite of the impossibility of certain performances which were formerly possible. But the new state of health is not the same as the old one ... Recovery is a newly achieved state of ordered functioning ... <u>a new individual norm</u>."

With this final emphasis, Goldstein affirms that the *new* norm, like the old one, must be an individual one and nothing imposed from without – based on ordered activities satisfying to the individual's essential nature – even if a portion of this 'essence' may have permanently lost its capacity for a full, undefective and ordered expression.

Life Medicine, like the reflections on health and illness that form part of the 'existential neurology' of Goldstein, also affirms the significance of *free choice* on the part of the patient. Thus there may be a situation in which a patient must freely decide whether and to what extent to *either* limit his or her existing life world and its ordered activities in the face of particular limits to their capacities *or* to continue to engage in these activities as before despite the pain or suffering that accompanies them (for example by staying in an over-demanding job).

Whatever the patient decides – with the potential help, encouragement and counselling of the physician as 'life doctor' – the outcome is a way in which the patient freely decides to adapt his or her environment or milieu to his own needs and desires – rather than being forced to adapt *to* them.

Recognising this, we have immediately transcended the one-sided Darwinian notion that organisms survive and thrive solely by *adapting to their environment* – rather than *by adapting that environment* – their life world – in a way that best serves their essential health and well-being.

This is also significant given that most people live in *two* environments or 'life worlds'. One is a 'negative environment' in which social structures and economic conditions actually and constantly deprive individuals of potentials for healthy self-actualisation and instead overload them with demands unrelated to these potentials – often to the point where they cannot 'cope' with these demands or the lack of fulfilment they get from meeting them. As a result people get ill simply by virtue of adapting to a fundamentally unhealthy or sick social-economic environment – and are medically treated simply to restore their capacity to function economically in a way that serves that environment.

The other environment is whatever 'positive' environment, life world or milieu individuals are able to forge for themselves within or outside their 'negative' environment. This positive environment is one that genuinely serves the individual's need to take time, not just for rest, recuperation or distraction from the ills and illnesses induced by their negative environment, but also and above all for activities that serve their positive self-actualisation, and with it their essential *life health* – something that has nothing to do with so-called 'healthy lifestyles'.

Reference: Goldstein, Kurt *The Organism*

Life, Death and 'Terminal Illness'

"The name of the bow is life. Its work is death."
Heraclitus

The Greek word for 'life' (*bios*) also means 'bow'. Yet the apparent truism that life is a span of time drawn out, like the string of a bow, between birth and death, and that the very body that sustains our life will eventually also 'work' our death is one that most people would like to forget. Their belief in biological medicine is not just rooted in a quasi-religious respect for the authority of modern science and technology and its medical application. In many cases, it is also rooted in the false belief that birth and death are the alpha and omega of our existence as such i.e. that death brings a final end to our lives, to our consciousness – indeed to our very being – rather than releasing us, like a bow releases an arrow, into different and broader dimensions of existence, consciousness and life. This belief in turn is linked to the modern scientific notion that consciousness is a mere product or property of our bodies and brains – a notion that is actually quite illogical. For given that we only *know* we exist or have a body through a (conscious) *awareness* of being and of having a body, to reduce this *awareness* of our bodies to some product or property *of* our bodies, is like reducing our entire *dream awareness* to the product or property of some particular thing we are aware of dreaming.

As for what we think of as our bodies themselves, there is not an atom in them that does not itself 'survive' the disintegration of the human organism – or is not imbued with its own consciousness. Yet the body that concerns us here is not what we think of as our 'mortal' or 'physical' body but rather what in Life Medicine goes by the name of the 'lived' or 'felt body '. Since this body is essentially nothing but a *body of consciousness*, a distinct 'psychic body' or 'soul body', it cannot but survive the disintegration of our physical body and its soul – made up of atomic and molecular consciousness.

For centuries however, the understanding that the soul itself has its own innate bodily shape and form – its *own* body – has been surrendered to a false separation of 'body' and 'mind' – or 'body' and 'soul'. Paradoxically therefore, whereas most people believe that the possibility of life after death depends on the body and soul being separate entities, in a sense the very opposite is the case – the soul survives death by virtue of having its own body. Proof of the 'existence' of such a body requires no supposedly 'scientific' form of experimentation or evidence, nor even the experience of dreaming or so-called 'out of body' states in which we inhabit another, entirely subjective body. For in reality this felt body or 'soul body' – the body as we subjectively feel and experience it – is and can be the *only body* that we ever experience. Its existence is therefore 'empirically' self-evident and not an hypothesis to be proven.

Even putting such philosophical arguments aside however, the fact remains that the very *belief* that death marks the ultimate terminus or end point of our being and consciousness is in many cases a principal reason why so many people with actual or potentially 'terminal' illnesses resort to biomedical treatments. For if death truly is the terminal point of our existence, then it will seem to them that their 'life' depends on such treatments, i.e. life and being *as such* and not just their existence in *this life*. So for them any medical means of forestalling death or extending their current life is understandably attractive to them – even if it comes at the expense of further *weakening* their own bodies through treatments such as invasive surgery, radiotherapy or chemotherapy, and/or severely reducing their quality of life through other side effects of such treatments.

178

That is why another important role of the Life Doctor is to help patients come to more deeply considered decisions about whether or not to accept the forms of biomedical treatment that may be recommended to them – often with considerable pressure. Above all, however, the Life Doctor must be able to reassure the patient with *absolute personal and philosophical conviction* that *no one* – whether seemingly healthy or severely ill – dies before they are inwardly ready to die for some reason connected with their current life and existence in all its dimensions – and not just the life of 'the body' as biological medicine understands it.

"... no person dies ahead of his or her time. The individual chooses the time of death. It is true however, that many cancers and conditions such as AIDS result because the immunity system has been so tampered with that the body has not been allowed to follow through with its own balancing act."

"Again, however, no individual dies of cancer or AIDS, or any other condition, until they themselves have set the time."

Seth, in *The Way Toward Health* (see appendix 6)

Seth also adds the following insights, all of which form part of the philosophical framework of Life Medicine and Life Doctoring:

"People with life-threatening diseases ... often feel that further growth, development, or expansion are highly difficult, if not impossible to achieve at a certain point in their lives. Often there are complicated family relationships that the person does not know how to handle ... In all cases, however, the need for value fulfilment, expression, and creativity are so important to life that when these are threatened, life itself is at least momentarily weakened. Innately, each person does realise that there is life after death, and in some instances such people realise that it is indeed time to move to another level of reality, to die and set out again with another brand new world ... Often, seriously ill people quite clearly recognise such feelings but they have been taught not to speak of them. The desire to die is considered cowardly, even evil, by some religions – and yet behind that desire lies all of the vitality of the will to life, which may already be seeking new avenues of expression and meaning."

An important role of the Life Doctor in relation to so-called 'terminal illness' should therefore be to question how the very term 'terminal' is understood by the patient – in other words whether they themselves see death as an absolute termination of their being or can understand it as a return and transition of the soul to a "brand new world", i.e. a different dimension of consciousness in which possibilities of expression, growth and development frustrated in their current life and world might be fulfilled. For behind the 'will to die' do not necessarily lie 'suicidal' impulses in the way they are ordinarily understood – as the expression of a desire to annihilate the self. Such impulses may also arise from a conscious or unconscious recognition of what the world to come offers the self in terms of greater fulfilment. This recognition is important in another way too – since many suicides would be avoided were the individual to realise that death does *not* bring an end to their life – or to important challenges not met within it.

As Seth points out, it is a scientific dogma "...that life is meaningless, that it has no purpose, and that its multitudinous parts fell together through the workings of chance alone..." adding that "such dogma is far more religious than scientific, for it also expects to be believed without proof, on faith alone. All of life is seen as heading for extinction in any case. The entire concept of a soul, life after death, or even life from one generation to the next, becomes doubtful, to say the least ... In such a philosophical world it would seem that man has no power at all... those concepts can have a hand in the development of would-be suicides, particularly of a young age, for they seem to effectively block a future."

This question of 'life after death' then is by no means 'merely' metaphysical or philosophical, for every individual bears within them a set of philosophical beliefs or assumptions with a profound bearing on their relation not just to health and illness, but to the relation of medicine to life and death.

"There are those who come down with one serious disease – say heart trouble – who are cured through a heart transplant or other medical procedure, only to fall prey to another, seemingly unrelated disease, such as cancer. It would relieve the minds of family and friends, however if they understood that the individual involved did not 'fall prey' to the disease, and that he or she was not a victim in usual terms ... This does not mean that anyone consciously decides to get such-and-such a disease, but it does mean that some people instinctively realise that their own development does now demand another new framework of existence."

"Much loneliness results when people who know they are going to die feel unable to communicate with loved ones for fear of hurting their feelings. Still other kinds of individuals will live long productive lives even while their physical mobility or health is most severely impaired. They will still feel that they had work to do, or that they were needed ..."

Specifically with regard to cancer, Seth comments that:

"Many cancer patients have martyr-like characteristics, often putting up with undesirable situations or conditions for years. They feel powerless, unable to change, yet unwilling to stay in the same position. The most important point is to arouse such a person's belief in his or her strength and power. In many instances these people shrug their shoulders, saying "What will happen, will happen," but they do not physically struggle against their [life] situation."

"It is ... vital that these patients are not overly medicated, for oftentimes the side effects of some cancer-eradicating drugs are dangerous in themselves. There has been some success with people who imagine that the cancer is instead some hated enemy or monster or foe, which is then banished with mental mock battles over a period of time. While the technique does have its advantages, it also pits one portion of the self against the other." [my stress]

"Cancer patients most usually feel an inner impatience as they sense their own need for future expansion and development, only to feel it thwarted." [my stress]

"Again, we cannot generalise overmuch, but many persons *know quite well that they are not sure whether they want to live or die.* The overabundance of cancer cells represents nevertheless the need for expression and expansion – the only arena left open – or so it would seem."

(from *The Way Toward Health*, by Jane Roberts)

The phrases I have italicised above offer important insights that Life Doctoring for patients with potentially terminal illnesses needs to take account of.

On the one hand, they affirm the general understanding of Life Medicine that in seeking to 'fight', 'conquer' or 'get rid of' an illness, one is effectively trying to fight, conquer or get rid of a vital part of ourselves – a part that is showing us how 'sick' or ill-at-ease we are with our lives or way of living – and that in a very specific way for which the timing and specific nature of our illness will always offer us clear clues.

On the other hand, they return us again to fundamental issues of life and death – or rather beliefs regarding them. For, if death is seen as the final end of life and being, then there might not only be an understandable *impatience* both to 'cure' any disease we believe can or will kill us – regardless of our will to live – but perhaps also an impatience to 'live life to the full' in whatever limited period of time we believe (or are led to believe) we still have. This again is understandable, and yet there is also the possibility that this intense impatience to 'make the best use' of our remaining years or 'live them to the full' (whether we are healthy or ill) may be a concealed expression of a still unacknowledged *will to die* – expressed through an impatient desire to get through these years not just as intensely but also as *quickly* as possible.

Another important key to Life Doctoring for 'life-threatening' illness is therefore *patience as such*. That is because for whatever reasons and in whatever ways an individual may have become or continues to remain 'a patient' – this may be a result either of them being *too patient* with their life circumstances or too *impatient* to deal with them except through illness, biomedical treatments – or even an exaggerated 'will to live'. For through this will to live some 'patients' *may* be seeking to impatiently hide from a still unacknowledged 'will to die' – or to impatiently *deny* any remaining inner conflict between their will to live and their will to die. This dilemma becomes even more charged as a 'life or death issue' if a patient is or feels pressured to quickly decide for example, whether to *immediately accept* potentially dangerous forms of biomedical testing and treatment – or simply *to be patient* – not just to 'wait and see' but to give themselves time to see more deeply into themselves, their life and their illness. At such times it might well be of great importance for 'the patient' to heed the words of Martin Heidegger: *"Patience is the truly human mode of being."*

Life Medicine and the Secret of Longevity

'Longevity' is usually understood as living for a long time. Yet one can live for a 100 years or more and still lead a life dominated by 'time poverty' and/or lacking in 'quality time'. And being too busy to experience life in all its richness, depth and fullness – and to draw meaning and fulfilment from it – is itself a major cause of illness. In contrast to the association of 'life' itself with permanent activity and 'busy-ness', Life Medicine recognises that the true 'length' of our lives has less to do with the mere quantity of years we live than with the quality and extent of the time we *take for ourselves* and others whilst living them. Indeed *taking time* – by which I mean 'taking our own time' – is the true secret of health and longevity in *every sense* – both qualitative and quantitative. A life lived more slowly – given more time – is both a richer and a longer life. The key to this in turn is *making time* or *taking time* for ourselves, for others – and for all the things listed below – and many more:

Taking time to feel and be more aware of our bodies *all the time* – and not just when we are ill.

Taking time to feel and be more aware of our bodies *as a whole* – and not the just the parts of them we are using or feeling *at any given time.*

Taking time to be aware of our *breathing* – and to consciously breathe more slowly.

Taking time to be more aware of our *speaking* – and to consciously speak more slowly.

Taking time to feel our thoughts and feelings more deeply *before* we speak them.

Taking time to feel and adjust our posture and to relax our muscles *before* speaking or moving.

Taking time to allow longer intervals of silence in communication – intervals in which we take all the time we need to silently take in and digest what another person has said *before* reacting to it.

Taking time to premeditate any activities *before* we engage in them, to choose and *time* our actions and interactions in a way that feels right in our bodies – neither needlessly rushing or delaying them – and *never* just 'going from one thing to another' in time.

Taking time to *pause* and *stop time* – to create 'breathing spaces' between *every single* interaction, task or activity we engage in – time to rest from them, to recollect, digest and process our experience of them, to feel for deeper layers of meaning in them – and let fresh insights arise from them.

Taking time to feel for and return to a place of deep inner stillness and silence within us before our next actions or words – so that we act and speak from that place of inner stillness and silence.

Taking time to 'open ourselves' bodily – to feel and take in the entire space around our bodies.

Taking time to 'ground ourselves' bodily – to feel the ground beneath our feet and our entire lower body below the waist.

Taking time to 'centre' both ourselves and our breathing in our true spiritual and physical centre of gravity – our lower abdomen – using *only* our abdominal muscles to breathe and feeling the inner space of the abdomen as the true seat and centre of both our body and self.

Taking time to 'body' what we feel before expressing or acting on our feelings – for example to find a tone of voice, facial expression or look in our eyes that truly fits the way we feel inside.

Taking time to make wordless feeling contact with others before speaking with them – to feel and take another person in as 'some body' and not just an 'other mind' or 'talking head'.

Taking time to 'come to our senses' – using our bodies to experience more vividly and intensely the immediate sensory and sensuous dimension of every encounter or experience, person or place, thought or emotion, situation or state of being.

Taking time to be with and 'bear with' ourselves and others in 'pregnant silence' – thus allowing new ways of feeling ourselves and relating to others – a new 'inner bearing' – to be born from that pregnant silence.

Taking time in all these ways – not just to *slow down* but also to *savour* time – to let every single experienced life activity, event or encounter *linger on* in our bodies and *fill them* with felt and *living meaning*.

Taking time in this way to experience true inner 'fulfillment' in life – rather than trying to just 'lead a full life'.

Taking time to be truly *patient* with our bodies, our feelings and our lives – and in this way both deepen and stretch out *time itself* – rather than becoming 'a patient' or seeking to 'extend' our life.

'The Secret of Longevity' – taking more time in one's life to be more aware of *time itself* – and to *linger* in a bodily way with all that occurs within it.

Distinctions Central to Life Medicine

Basic Distinctions

Life Medicine is rooted in a number of new and fundamental distinctions.

1. Between feeling ill and 'getting ill'.

2. Between feeling ill-at-ease with one's life and being 'ill'.

3. Between the particular life meaning of an illness for the individual and its biological 'causes'.

4. Between our subjectively 'felt body' or 'lived body' and the 'clinical body' or 'physical' body.

5. Between the body as an embodiment of the human *being* and the body as a biological *machine*.

6. Between our subjectively felt sense of bodily 'dis-ease' and an 'objective' bio-medically diagnosed 'disease'.

7. Between seeing the patient's life problem *as their illness* and seeing the patient's illness as the symptom of a *life problem*.

8. Between talking to a doctor *because* one is ill and getting ill in order to talk to a doctor.

9. Between seeing illness itself *as a symptom* and seeing symptoms only as possible *signs of an illness*.

10. Between knowing that one may die *by means* of an illness and believing that one dies simply 'from' an illness.

11. Between *meditating* an illness to heal one's life and *medicating* an illness to heal one's body.

12. Between seeing a patent's illness as something to be cured and understanding that *the illness is there to cure the patient* – to help them to heal and transform their lives.

Table of Differences:
Biological Medicine versus Life Medicine

Assumptions of Biological Medicine	Basic Principles of Life Medicine
The purpose of medicine is to *cure the illness*.	The purpose of illness is to *cure the patient.*
The illness is the enemy.	The illness is the cure.
Health is 'good'. Illness is 'bad'.	Illness is part of a healthy life, just as dealing with life-problems is.
Health and illness are opposites.	Illness is a natural part of a healthy life.
The *human body* can be separated from the life of the individual *human being*.	The human body is a *living embodiment* of the individual human being.
The patient's life problem is their *illness* and its symptoms.	The patient's illness is the symptom of a *life problem*.
Illnesses are *things* that we 'get' or 'have'.	Illnesses are natural life and learning *processes*.
Illnesses have 'causes' but no *life meaning* – aside from interfering with our lives and thus requiring treatment.	Illnesses have *life meanings* – symbolising, and thus helping us explore important life questions.

A somatic symptom is a diagnostic 'sign' of a bodily disease.	A symptom is a somatic *symbol* of a felt *dis-ease*
Diagnosis identifies *independent disease entities* in the body and thus guides treatment.	There are *no such things* as disease entities separable from the body and life of the individual as whole.
Illness can be life-threatening and thus a cause of death. People die *from* illness if they are untreated or incurable.	People die *through* illnesses and not 'from' or 'of' them – and do so only if they are *ready to die*.
The aim of medicine is to 'cure' or rid ourselves of an illness.	The illness itself is the potential 'cure' – helping to heal or 'make whole' our self.
Illness is an *attack* by 'foreign bodies' or 'non-self' organisms such as viruses or mutated cells.	Illness is a form of *pregnancy* – the bodily expression of unborn aspects of our self as a whole.
Medicine is *war* against disease – helping our bodies to 'fight' disease.	Medicine is *midwifery* – helping us to give birth to a new sense of self.
Healing means bringing about changes *in our bodies.*	Healing means *letting our bodies change us* – our bodily sense of self.
Mind and body 'affect' one another though physiological processes.	Every bodily or somatic state *is* a state of consciousness – and vice versa.

Illness is the result of an *objective* biological process occurring in the *physical body*	Illness is the result of changes occurring in our subjective or *felt body* – which is also our bodily identity, our 'body self'.
Feeling ill results from 'getting ill' with some objective physical 'disease'.	'Getting ill' results from feeling ill – from a subjectively felt *dis-ease*.
The way we feel our bodies – our inwardly felt body – is a subjective expression of the physical body.	The physical body is an outward expression of our subjective body – our inwardly felt body.
The aim of the physician is to help the patient to recover or 'feel themselves' again – to feel the same way they did before getting ill.	The aim of the physician is to help the patient to change – to feel a different self to the one they felt before getting ill.
The purpose of the physician-patient relationship is to heal the patient by diagnosing and treating their symptoms.	It is the *relationship itself* that is the chief healing factor, helping – or not helping – the patient to heal.
The health of the individual is an entirely private matter and a function of their bodies.	Individual health is an expression of the health of *human relations* in society. Sicknesses are sicknesses of relation.
Symptoms are caused by a *physical disease* or disorder in the *human body or brain*.	Both symptoms and their causes are the expression of a *felt dis-ease* of the individual *human being*.

Symptoms have bodily *causes*.	Symptoms are bodily *symbols*.
The human body is a *functioning biological machine*.	The human body is a *living biological language*.
We 'have' a body – a body which we can feel in different ways.	We do not 'have' a body. We *body* – *embodying* the way we feel.
Health is our capacity to maintain a *fully functioning* body and mind, no matter how sick the society in which we live.	Health is our capacity to *fully embody* and *fulfil* our values and potentials as individual human beings.
Every patient's illness is just an individual 'case' of a generic disease.	Every patient's illness is a unique expression of their individuality.
Medical science is based on 'proven facts', such as the way the immune system functions.	Modern medicine is based on *linguistic metaphors* – such as the *military* metaphor of immune 'defences'.
Most medical research is 'neutral' and 'objective'.	Most medical research is profit driven and biased by corporate funding.
Most medications are scientifically trialled and tested to show their effectiveness and safety.	Most medications are little more effective than placebos, whilst often producing severe or even life-threatening side effects.

Modern biomedical treatments of illness save countless lives and are therefore indispensable.	Statistics from recognised medical journals in the U.S.A. show that biomedical treatments are themselves *the third principal cause of death* after cancer and heart disease – if not *the* leading cause of death as well as countless *iatrogenic* (medically induced) illnesses and symptoms.
Inner well-being is an expression of the health of the body.	The health of the body is an expression of inner well-being.

Life Medicine and 'Alternative Medicine'

One of the principal attractions of 'alternative' forms of medicine is that its practitioners tend to give a lot more time to their patients than doctors– at least in the initial consultation – and to ask questions about their lives and life situation as a whole of a sort that biomedical doctors have no time for or see no point in. All the more disappointing then, that such initial consultations usually prove to be a mere *prelude* to a procedure identical in principle to that of any biomedical doctor i.e. internally framing and 'diagnosing' the patient's bodily symptoms in terms of an unquestioned body of knowledge (for example homeopathy or Traditional Chinese Medicine) and then prescribing some form of pre-given remedy or engaging in some form of pre-prescribed alternative 'treatment' – all in a way that the practitioner has been *taught* is appropriate to the patient's condition according to their training – and which therefore demands of them no further or deeper thought.

The effectiveness of the alternative remedies or treatments is in large part due to the *relationship* of trust established between practitioner and patient and to their joint *belief* in the rationale and efficacy of whatever remedy or operational procedure (for example a selected acupunctural procedure) is prescribed. Belief and trust are the real foundation of the so-called 'placebo effect' – though this is a no less important factor in the efficacy of much orthodox biomedical practice than it is in the practice of alternative medicine. For even so-called random double-blind drug trials designed to exclude subjective or observational bias on the part of *both* patient and researcher assume in advance that the patient's own body is *not itself aware* of whether it has been given a 'placebo' or a complex pharmaceutical drug even though the latter is bound to be registered and reacted to by the body and registered by the patient in one way or another.

The term 'alternative medicine' belongs to a variety of so-called approaches to medicine regarded as 'holistic' – that claim to 'treat' the person and not just the disease, i.e. the human being as a 'whole' and not just their body. Yet the very language of medicine and of holistic healing – in particular the use of the little word 'and' in stock phrases such as 'mind *and* body', 'body *and* soul' or 'body, mind *and* spirit' effectively reduces the human being to a mere assemblage of separate parts. In this way holistic medicine is again, no different in essence from biological medicine – with which it also shares the *same basic aim* of seeking 'causes' and 'cures' for illness rather than exploring its life meaning for the patient. Indeed the term 'holistic healing' does not even make linguistic sense, for it constitutes what is called a pleonasm like 'black darkness'. That is because the words 'whole' and 'holistic' actually share many of the same roots as the word 'healing' itself – for example the Middle English *hole/hoole* and *hāl* from which the words 'hail' – meaning 'be blessed with long life' – 'hale' and 'healthy' are derived. In its linguistic roots, therefore, the phrase 'holistic healing' means nothing more than 'healing which makes healthy'.

On the other hand, alternative methods of healing such as acupressure, acupuncture and different types of massage can certainly be understood as stimulating a type of healing inter-cellular communication between different organs and parts of the body – not through the flow of any 'thing' that might be called 'energy' but rather in the form of breath or air-like flows of atomic, molecular and cellular awareness. Understanding such flows in this way can help bring us closer to essence of what is called 'Alternative Medicine' and its distinction from both Biological Medicine and Life Medicine – namely that it works *neither* through the so-called 'physical body' nor through any form of 'energy body' but rather through that bounded portion of our larger 'body of feeling' awareness' or 'lived body' that can be called the 'physical soul'.

Understood in this way, alternative medicine in all its forms may indeed be effective in ameliorating or working on *symptoms* in a way that does not rely on conventional forms of biomedical testing and treatment. Yet even though biomedicine recognises neither a psychical 'body of awareness' nor a 'physical soul' made up of organised and organising patterns of atomic, molecular and cellular awareness, the 'effectiveness' of alternative medicine tends to be assessed – even by its own practitioners – *in exactly the same terms as biomedicine*. That is why this 'effectiveness' can and often is disputed or dismissed on the basis of the purely statistical or so-called 'evidence-based' criteria of biomedical science and research, which (like alternative medicine) singularly fails to research and assess what is most important of all and yet not something *measurable* in principle – namely the individual *life meaning* of a given symptom or illness for a patient as opposed to its supposedly universal 'causes' or 'cures' and the impersonal, statistical 'evidence' on which they are based.

Biomedicine and alternative medicine differ essentially only in the *language* they use to describe such 'causes' and in the 'cures' they offer. Thus whereas a biomedical practitioner may seek the causes of a disease in our genes or in organic disorders, a practitioner of alternative medicine may seek them in the form of 'blockages' in 'energy flows', an imbalance of so-called 'energy centres' or 'chakras', a lack of specific vitamins or nutrients, or a surfeit of 'bad' ones. And whereas a biomedical practitioner may prescribe a pharmaceutical drug with serious side effects or invasive and potentially dangerous operative surgery as a 'cure', the alternative practitioner merely offers a different form of 'cure' in the form, say, of a natural herb or a safer type of treatment procedure such as massage or acupuncture. The use of both may, like pharmaceutical drugs, either serve as a placebo and/or have very genuine effects on what I call the 'physical soul'.

And yet, as I repeatedly emphasise, unlike 'alternative' or 'complementary' medicine, the focus of Life Medicine is neither on the physical soul or 'body consciousness' (i.e. the innate consciousness of our cells and tissues) and nor, like mainstream Biological Medicine, is its focus on the 'physical body' – which is nothing but the physical soul as perceived from the outside. Yet the physical soul is, again, but one portion of the lived body or soul body as a whole. Hence if *only* the patient's body consciousness or physical soul is treated by whatever means – including those of 'alternative medicine' – then, despite all talk of treating the 'whole person' or of 'holistic forms' of medicine uniting 'body and soul', the patient's larger soul and its body, their body of feeling awareness, remains unseen and unsensed.

In this sense the life of the human being and human body as a whole – their soul – is still ignored and left out of the picture even in alternative medicine. That is why, just as is the case in biological medicine (and no matter how more empathic, personable' or 'person-centred' the 'alternative' or 'complementary' practitioner may be) the patient may be left feeling dis-ensouled. For whether in the form of homeopathic prescriptions, herbal remedies, touch therapies or acupuncture, the patient still ends up being given essentially *impersonal* forms of treatment, often also in a quasi-clinical setting and manner. Many alternative practitioners therefore effectively treat their patient, like biomedicine, merely as 'some body' – and not at all as a unique, living, breathing and embodied soul – one with a soul life and a soul body that extends far beyond the boundaries of the flesh and embraces their entire life world. Then again, the patient as a 'person' is but one face of their soul. The patient's larger soul life and life world however – and *its* relation to their illness – is something that not even the most detailed medical history can offer a practitioner of any sort the slightest clues to – unless, as in the practice of Life Medicine, it is 'complemented' by also taking a detailed *life* history of the patient.

Finally, treating *only* the physical soul of a patient – whether through standard pharmaceutical drugs or through herbal remedies, touch therapies or 'alternative medicine' of *any* sort – carries its own dangers. For *any* externally induced alterations to the physical soul can have deep and even traumatic effects on the psyche and lived body of the patient as a whole – effects which practitioners of alternative or 'holistic' medicine who are untrained in any form psychotherapy or psychological counselling are ill-equipped to deal with.

Etymological note 1 – on the terms 'whole' and 'heal'

It is a common but false belief that the root meaning of the verb 'to heal' is to 'make whole'. It is true that the word *holistic* comes from the Greek *holos* meaning entire or 'whole'. The word w*hole* itself however, comes from Middle English *hole/hoole or hāl* – meaning not only 'healthy' but also 'sound' – as in the German words *Hall* ('echoing sound') and *gesund* – 'healthy' – but also in the sense of a gathering (*ge-*) of 'sound' (-*sund*) as in *a hall* – German *Halle*. A hall is a place of shelter but one that also echoes, reverberates and resounds (German *hallen*).

All these English and Germanic words connected with what is 'whole', 'hale' or 'healthy' are thus also intimately related to the German words *heilig/das Heilige* and their English equivalents – *holy* and *the holy* – which in turn refer not just to what is divine or sacred, but also and at the same time that which silently *sounds and resounds* through all that is. Hence the English *hale* and German *heil*, to be in 'sound' health. Hence also the German greeting *Heil!* and English *hail!* – greeting sounds that offer a divine blessing, grant good fortune, salvation and wish the other a long life – and that are echoed today in the everyday greeting words *hello* (English) and *hallo* (German).

The German verb *heilen* and English *to heal* – originally meaning to 'protect', 'redeem' or 'save', are all rooted in the Germanic *hailaz* – meaning a sounded magical or sacred blessing, and go back to the Indo-European *kail.* The opposite of all that is sound and hale is what in German is called *das Unheil* – usually translated as 'misfortune', 'calamity', 'catastrophe' or 'disaster'. Yet what sort of 'calamity' or 'catastrophe' is meant here? One that merely causes or results from some sort of accidental misfortune – as illness or ill-health is thought to do. Surely not, since the word *Unheil* has related senses of something being not only unhealthy or unholy but also *unsound.* 'To heal' then, is not simply to restore health in the sense of curing or eliminating a disease but rather to restore the essence of health as 'soundness' or *Ge-sundheit* – to restore *resonance.* For where there is no longer any felt sense of resonance with another human being, how can the human being once again be brought into resonance with the holy – that which shelters and speaks to all beings within the cosmos, understood as a 'hall' or 'house' of God? That is why holy caves and temples were the first places people went to for 'healing '. It is also why the vocations of 'holy man', 'shaman' or 'priest' on the one hand – guardian of a holy cave, hall or temple – and healer on the other, were originally one. The holy man (or woman) was also a human being who effectively worked their capacity (*energein*) to use *holy* sounds and speech in the form of syllables, spells, mantras or prayers to heal – these being sounds and speech *in resonance* with the divine soul of the human being.

The Anatomy & Physiology of the Lived Body

Life Doctoring is based on a quite different understanding of anatomy and physiology than that which is taken as standard by biological medicine - and also by some forms of 'alternative medicine'. That is because Life Medicine understands the body essentially as a body of feeling awareness or soul, and the felt surface of the body as we perceive it from the outside – the so-called physical body' - as essentially nothing more than a boundary uniting and distinguishing two *fields* of awareness. These two fields are:

1. an outer field of awareness encompassing and embracing the entire life *world* of the individual and all they experience within it including both things and other people.
2. an inner field of awareness consisting not of fleshly tissue and organs but of hollow spaces of awareness felt within the regions of the head, chest or heart, and abdomen or 'hara' (Japanese) respectively.

Part of both the training and work of the Life Doctor consists in cultivating their own and their patients' ability to sense these outer and inner spaces or fields of feeling awareness, and to experience the latter as a singular inner space of feeling awareness allowing it to flow and centre itself freely in the regions of 'head, heart and hara'.

Life Medicine also distinguishes between:

1. the lived body as a whole, which embraces *both* fields of feeling awareness or 'soul'.
2. that portion of its inner field which takes the form of the 'body consciousness' or 'physical soul' – composed of those organising patterns of molecular and cellular awareness which are perceived from the outside (and within the outer field of any individual's awareness) in the form of the 'physical body'.

3. The atomic, molecular and, in the case of plants and animals, the cellular awareness which make up the physical soul of all perceived phenomena within the outer field of any individuals awareness, i.e. within their experienced life world or environment.

Finally, Life Medicine distinguishes between physiological functions and processes generally seen as belonging to the physical body and its organs – such as respiration, ingestion digestion and metabolisation of food – and the basic function of the lived body – namely to breathe in, digest and metabolise their lived subjective *experience* of themselves, other people and the world around them. It is these basic functions (or dysfunctions) of awareness that manifest in 'organic' physiological functions or dysfunctions – and not the other way round. Similarly it is patterns, tones, intensities and intents arising from feeling awareness that manifest as the sensed tone and motility of tissue and organs, muscular tonus and patterns of muscular tensioning and movement.

A basic motto of Life Medicine is that we are as much aware of our 'self' as a whole – our soul – as we are aware of our body as a whole - including both its outer field and all the inwardly felt regions or spaces *of* awareness that form part of its 'inner field'.

As well as their capacity to directly see into and sense the tones of feeling awareness pervading the inner head, chest and abdominal spaces of the patient's lived body, the advanced Life Doctor can also use their own lived body to sense various other critical features of patient's own felt or lived body as a whole.

That is also why, in addition to biographical questioning (see *What Most Doctors Don't Ask*) and in order to raise their own awareness of these features, questions of a very different sort tend also to be put to the patient during initial Life Doctoring consultations. For example:

1. To what degree, on a scale of 1 to 10, can you inwardly feel your body as a whole – from top to toe – including not just your head or upper body, but your entire lower body below the waist, including your legs and reaching down to the soles of your feet?

2. To what extent, on a scale of 1 to 10, are you aware of the entire surface skin and musculature of your upper body – including the surface skin and musculature of your face and eyes, of the surface of your entire head – top, front, back and sides, and of your trunk – front, back and sides?

3. To what extent can you feel the sensed inwardness of your felt body surface – in particular those of your head, chest and abdomen - as part of a 'body without organs' i.e. as hollow spaces filled with nothing but feeling awareness or 'soul'.

4. To what extent, on a scale of 1-10 do you feel you are as much aware of your entire lower body below the waist as you are of your head, chest and upper body?

5. On an imaginary vertical line extending from the crown of your head to the soles of your feet, point to where you feel your *breathing* is centred.

6. On the same imaginary line point to where you feel your *awareness* is centred.

7. To what degree do you feel you can lower the centre of (a) your awareness and (b) your breathing, from a point in the inner region of your head or chest or belly to one in the region of your lower abdomen. Use your hand to point to the lowest point at which your can feel your awareness and your breathing centred.

8. Using your arms or hands, indicate both the size of any clear and hollow inner space or spaces of awareness you feel enclosed by your body surface and also *where* you feel that space or those spaces – whether just in your head, your upper body, or in your trunk as a whole including your abdomen.

9. To what extent, on a scale of 1-10, do you feel yourself and your awareness to be contained or encapsulated by your body surface, as if you were simply looking out at the world through 'the peepholes of the senses' – rather than actually sensing, encompassing and embracing that world in a larger more spacious *field* of awareness?

10. To what degree, on a scale of 1 to 10, do you feel your body surface to be sensitive to and aware of the entire space surrounding you in this room and all it contains?

11. Using your arms to indicate to what extent you feel your awareness extending into space in a way that reaches beyond the boundaries of your fleshly skin.

The answers sensed and given to these questions tell the Life Doctor about the specific 'anatomy' of the patient's lived body, as well as providing suggestive keys to the patient about what it means to cultivate feeling awareness of their lived body as a whole – a body which is not enclosed or bounded by one's skin but embraces all the spaces within *and* around it. Such whole-body awareness is a foundation for well-being as well as for the patient's own capacity for self-doctoring. The questions above also provide a foundation for teaching the patient to engage in four basic movements or motions of awareness that are central to both sustaining whole-body awareness. These basic motions of awareness are:

1. **Grounding** – recovering and sustaining whole-body awareness – in particular through heightened awareness of one's entire *lower body* below the waist as well as one's head and upper body.

2. **Centering** – learning to seat or centre both one's *breathing* and one's very *sense of self* within the felt inner space of the lower abdomen: this being that spiritual and physical centre of gravity of the human being known as *hara* in traditional Japanese culture, but generally ignored

in cultures that see human life only as an interplay of 'head' and 'heart'.

3. **Unifying** – feeling the hollow inwardness of one's head, chest ('heart') and abdominal region ('hara') as a singular and unified space of feeling awareness 1 – and one within which our awareness, like our breathing, can also be allowed to freely flow and centre itself in different regions and at different points.

4. **Opening** – using one's upper body surface to sense the entire space surrounding one's body as a whole and all other bodies within that space. In this way coming to experience one's entire body surface as 'all eye' and as a totally porous membrane – one through which one can experience oneself as literally *breathing in* one's *awareness* of the light and space around one.

5. **Facing** – giving form to a felt bodily sense of dis-ease through the look in one's face and eyes, thereby both intensifying that sense of dis-ease and also coming to feel it as an all-pervasive state of consciousness i.e. an underlying mood, tone or texture of feeling awareness or soul that can be *expressively embodied* – rather than 'somatised' in the form of one or more localised bodily sensations, symptoms or organic disorders.

References:

Wilberg, Peter *Head, Heart and Hara, the Soul Centres of West and East* New Gnosis Publications, 2003 Wilberg, Peter *The Little Book of Hara* (Kindle e-book)

Life Medicine and 'Energy Medicine'

"Science is the new religion."

Martin Heidegger

What might be called 'energeticism' has long become the new 'materialism' – an insight that nicely equates with Einstein's famous mathematical equation of energy and matter. Hence, in almost all 'alternative' or 'New Age' forms of healing that are offered in place of biological medicine, one word is *religiously* worshipped above all. This is the scientific-sounding word 'energy' – as used in the terms 'energy medicine' and 'energy body '. Through the use of the term energy, deference is made to a central term in the "new religion" of modern science – yet without any attempt to define or question what exactly is meant by this term – what 'energy' as such essentially *is*.

Behind this lack of basic questioning lies ignorance of both the linguistic and historic roots of the word 'energy' – for example the fact that the term 'energy' was first promoted in the 19th century by a group of well-known scientists called 'Energeticists' who wanted to place the term at the very top of the ladder of physical-scientific concepts.

"... the 'Energeticist Movement' associated with Wilhelm Ostwald around the turn of the 19th century advocated a World Government based on the use of 'energy' as the universal, unifying concept not only for all of physical science, but also for economics, psychology, sociology and the arts ... Not accidentally, the Kelvin-Helmholtz doctrine of 'energy' became a key feature of Anglo-American geopolitics, from the British launching of Middle East 'oil politics' at the beginning of the 20th century ... to a new Middle East war." from *The Difference between Dynamis and Energia* by Jonathan Tennenbaum

The fact remains however that the modern scientific concept of 'energy' *bears little relation* either to its roots in the Greek language *or* to the vocabulary of *any* ancient 'spiritual' or 'healing' tradition whatsoever, Eastern or Western.

For if we look at the original meaning of those Greek words from which the term 'energy' is derived, it make no sense to speak, for example of 'energy imbalances', or of *working* in any way 'on' or with our own or someone else's 'energy'. That is because one of the most basic root meanings of the Greek word *energeia* is purely and simply *'to be engaged in work'* or *'to be engaged in a work'* and consequently also *'to actualise something'.* So to speak of working 'with' or 'on' energy is tautological – meaning nothing more, in Greek terms, than 'working' with or on a 'work' one is engaged in.

Given its Western and *Greek* roots, the term 'energy' is *least of all* appropriate in translating Oriental terms such as *Chi*/QI or *Ki* that are so central to Chinese and Japanese forms of healing such as *Chi Gong* or *Reiki.* To speak of *Chi/Qi* or *Ki* as some sort of 'energy' flowing through the body (for example through so-called 'meridian' lines) also makes no linguistic sense, since the Oriental ideograms for words such as *Chi/Qi* and *Ki*, do *not* refer to any form or flow of 'energy' but rather, like the Sanskrit *prana* or the Greek *psyche* – to breath ('the breath of life'). What in Oriental or Orientally-derived healing traditions is translated as 'energy' can instead best be understood instead as essentially a breath or air-like flow of *awareness* – for example to a particular point or points in the body where pressure is applied or acupuncture needles are inserted.

Today however, no one even thinks of questioning the use of the now taken-for-granted and sacrosanct term 'energy ', the many varieties of 'energy medicine' in which it has become so central, or the way in which it is used to mistranslate terms derived from ancient healing traditions. In this way however, the misuse and overuse of the modern term 'energy' not only blocks all fresh exploration of the *root meanings* of terms derived from these traditions, but also prevents a deeper exploration of the *root experiences* from which they first arose. So even today's highly trained and qualified practitioners or 'Masters' of these traditions do not think of asking themselves from what sort of direct, inwardly felt experiences of the human body such traditions arose in the first place, i.e. *before* they were systematised into unquestioned bodies of knowledge and structured into fixed or ritualised healing procedures and practices. They do not ask themselves, for example, how and in what manner Indian and Chinese sages first came to subjectively and inwardly sense what later came to be called 'nadis', 'meridians' or 'acupuncture points'? Nor do they recognise the vast historic, linguistic, experiential and cultural gulf that separates the intellectual abstraction of different 'energies' from traditional Greek, Galenic and Islamic medicine : with its emphasis on four essential *fluids* or 'humors' (yellow and black bile, blood and phlegm), four fundamental qualities (wet, dry, warm and cold) and four basic moods or 'temperaments' – choleric, melancholic, sanguine and phlegmatic – all of which were inwardly *felt* as central in shaping human bodily *self-experience*.

"It is the great error of Western philosophers that they always regard the human body intellectually, from the outside, as though it were not indissolubly a part of the active self."

Sato Tsuji

The Western tendency to confuse our *subjective* and inwardly *felt* body with intellectual concepts of an objective, *quasi-physical* body persists through the modern concepts of an 'energy body'. As a result, the use of terms like 'energy medicine' continues to substitute for a new type of 'phenomenological' research – inner feeling research – into the real experiential roots and *essence* of many traditional forms of healing and their languages. Instead the term 'energy' is used to offer a seemingly authoritative, scientific-sounding and 'objective' account of what is essentially an inner, *subjective* body – our 'lived body' or 'body of feeling awareness'. The result is that no progress is made towards a *radical rethinking* of traditional healing systems and practices; 'radical' because it truly returns to the *roots* of those traditions – bodily, experiential, historical and linguistic.

So it is that what today is misleadingly called 'Energy Medicine' has become the pseudo-scientific New Age substitute for 'Existential Medicine' or 'Life Medicine'. Yet only the latter can be said to be truly 'holistic' and also in resonance with the different root meanings of the term 'energy'. That is because Life Medicine is based on the recognition that 'to heal' means to address the actually experienced *life* of the human being as a whole – and the way it does or does not work to *actualise* and fulfil the latent *capacities* or *potentials* of the individual – work or action which effectively actualises specific potentials or capacities being the essential meaning of the Greek verb *energein*.

'Life Medicine' therefore, most certainly does *not* constitute yet another of the countless forms of 'Energy Medicine' currently promoted on the ever-expanding marketplace of traditional or New Age medical practices. Similarly, a 'Life Doctor' is not simply some sort of practitioner of alternative medicine who has been indoctrinated through training in an alternative body of medical 'knowledge' but rather someone with a carefully cultivated capacity to directly sense and *resonate* with the *lived body* and *life* of the patient as a whole – and in this way come to understand the inner connections between their illness and their life.

As for those who claim that evidence for an 'energy body' exists by virtue of the ability of some people to perceive a colourful 'aura' around the 'physical body' – or even to photograph it through exotic equipment – this only goes to show their ignorance of the true nature of the inwardly felt or lived body as what I call a 'body of feeling awareness'. For those who only *see* what they think of as a multi-coloured 'energetic' aura show only their inability to directly sense and *feel* the many and varied colourations of awareness or 'mood colours' that make up our lived body – even though these can be sensed by *any human being* and not just by trained 'clairvoyants' or practitioners of 'colour healing '. And for a practitioner of 'colour healing' to have to rely on colour charts that 'explain' how *seeing* a particular colour such as red in someone's 'aura' might, for example, 'mean' that this person has 'anger' in them, only goes to show how little capacity that practitioner has to directly *sense* that anger – rather than interpreting it "intellectually" and "from the outside" as some type of negative 'energy'.

All well and good, some might say, but surely the term 'energy' has long since passed, not just into New Age language but into ordinary, everyday language too – and that in a way which we all understand from experience – as when we speak of 'lacking energy' or feeling 'energetic'. That precisely is the danger however – namely that as soon as a word such as 'energy' passes into common everyday usage, we assume there is some 'thing' it refers to, and do not stop to ask ourselves what exactly it *is* we understand by the word or what sort of experience it is that we use it to name.

If we would ask ourselves these questions however, we would find ourselves coming closer to the root Greek meaning of the word 'energy' – and cease to think of it as any sort of 'thing' at all. After all, what is a state of having more or less 'energy' than an *awareness* of a greater or lesser *potential* (Greek *dynamis*) to engage in 'action' or 'work' (*ergon*), in particular action or work of a sort which can bring something to actualisation (*energein*)?

What we call 'energy' then, is itself and essentially a dimension of *awareness* – a feeling awareness of a greater or lesser potentiality to be engaged in action or work (*energeia*) and not an awareness of any objective 'thing' or entity, scientific or spiritual.

Illness is often accompanied by a state of what we call fatigue or 'low energy', i.e. the feeling awareness of a reduced *potentiality* for action and work. This state may prompt or force us to suspend some or all action or work or bring to a halt a period of overactivity or overwork – instead bringing us to rest for a shorter or longer time in awareness as such – a meditative awareness from which in turn new and *different* potentialities for action may germinate within us. By limiting our potentiality for action or work therefore, 'low' energy may actually be doing us good – not only forcing us to rest but in this way giving ourselves time to meditate on our lives – something more healing than any form of treatment or 'energy medicine' designed simply and purely to quickly 'boost' or 'restore' our energy – our capacity for action – but without any healing process or insights having occurred or arisen in our awareness.

Rather than explaining it as something to do with 'energies' in either a modern-scientific or New Age sense, Life Medicine helps us to understand illness itself *as* 'energy' – but in the essential and root sense of this word: namely as a feeling awareness, experienced through a sense of 'dis-ease', of a *potentiality for change* that is seeking self-actualisation (*energein*) whether through clinical disease or through a new relation to action and work (*ergon*).

Etymological note 2
– on the Greek roots of the term 'energy'

What unites all the following Greek roots of the word 'energy' are meanings to do with action or work, potentialities for action and the actualisation of potentials through work or action.

The Greek *ergon* was used to refer to any type of work.

Energein meant action or work which results in actual or effective result.

Energeia refers to a state of 'being-in-action' or 'being engaged in work'. So again, to speak of working 'on' or 'with' a person's 'energy' amounts to saying you are acting or working on action or work. Aristotle also used the term *energeia* to refer to specific states of consciousness or qualities of awareness associated with 'being in action' or 'being engaged in effective work' – happiness for example. However he denied the possibility of self-actualising *potentiality* and reduced the meaning of *energeia* to 'actuality'.

The words *energes/energos* meant 'powerful' and were used to describe powerful siege weapons for example.

Energema refers to activity which is an expression or embodiment of a potential, 'capacity' or 'capability'. It also means simply a working 'operation' or 'procedure' such as those carried out in surgery – or acupuncture – so again it makes no sense of that procedure working with or 'on' 'energy'.

Energeitai refers in the New Testament to the working of divine or supernatural powers (*energemata*) through human action (New Testament).

Energoumene refers to action (such as prayer) set in operation and empowered by the divine (New Testament). *Energesen* to things *worked* or 'wrought' by God (Old Testament).

Life Medicine and 'Spiritual Healing' – The Man Who Didn't Want to See

No form of medicine can guarantee a 'cure' for any illness – not least one whose basic principle is that 'the illness is the cure'. The types of truly effective self-healing that Life Doctoring can aid in therefore also require a readiness on the part of the individual patient to alter deep-seated and fundamental *beliefs* about the nature of medicine, health, illness and healing – and to concentrate *primarily* on attaining insights into the meaning of their illness rather than seeking to get rid of it through either conventional or alternative forms of medical treatment. This readiness to alter basic beliefs and interest in understanding both themselves and their illness more deeply may not always be present in the patient. If they also lack experience of any form of inter-personal counselling or therapy – or even have a negative view of it – such a readiness and interest may also be difficult to cultivate. Nevertheless, the importance of the type of insight into the meaning of an individual's illness that Life Medicine offers can even be exemplified by precisely this kind of unready patient, unwilling to see or change their fixed beliefs.

Case Example 4

The patient had, since 2003, been suffering from progressively worsening vision due to a retinal detachment in both eyes. Still being able to read, though only with a magnifier and book rest and more slowly and not as easily as someone with healthy eyes, Life Doctoring was conducted on a correspondence basis.

The Life Doctor was first contacted by the patient by e-mail for three reasons. Firstly, because the patient had exhausted all options offered by conventional medicine, secondly, because out of despair the patient had sought out a spiritual healer and tried alternative methods of healing (one of which promised cellular regeneration of the retina) and, thirdly, because the patient saw in the Life Doctor someone who, as a practitioner of a new form of yoga, could help him as a spiritual teacher and healer on his spiritual 'quest'. This was a quest not just for 'enlightenment' but also to develop superhuman yogic powers or *siddhis* – including not only powers of levitation but also and above all the power to heal his eyes himself.

Below I cite two of his own descriptions of his sight disorder and its relation to both the 'spiritual quest' it triggered and his notion of 'spiritual healing '.

"Since 2003 I am on the spiritual path due to severe vision-problems (deterioration and detachment of retinas), which urged me to give up my career. I studied hundreds of spiritual books, I am initiated into Kriya-Yoga in the line of Paramahamsa Yogananda and Roy Eugene Davis; I follow now a Taoist Buddhist path (Cosmic Freedom Qigong) to heal my eyes (trips to a healer in Brazil, John of God, helped me to avoid becoming totally blind. Now in one eye the retina is partially detached, with one eye I can see 30 %."

"No doctor can help me anymore. I already had 13 surgeries (both eyes, I think 10 in the left, 3 in the right eye). In both eyes the vitreous body has been removed, silicone has been filled into the eyeball (to re-attach the retina) and has then been removed again. In the left eye the procedure has been repeated without any success. In both eyes I have artificial lenses, because the operations had damaged the natural lens. There is no effective treatment with conventional medicine any more, it is over since 2003. I really did everything what was possible; during one of the operations there was a problem with local anaesthetics and I felt every stitch of a needle in my left eye. I got some treatments with eye-laser, the first of which was so painful that my whole body was wet with sweat after treatment. I was in hell. Only my trips to Brazil to "John of God" had helped me a bit – my eye doctor (an internationally well-known expert) was astonished that I had not become totally blind in both eyes. She even told me to go to Brazil again! In 2003 I had already purchased a gun to commit suicide, but after my first trip to Brazil (April 2004) my condition improved and again I hoped for a healing. In Brazil I was very brave: John of God claims to be a medium for high Beings (King Salomon, Ignatius from Loyola …) who accomplishes spiritual operations through his body and I trusted him. I got a knife directly into the edge of my eyeball, hoping that his claims were true and they were. I had nothing to lose. There is no apparent other illness in my physical body, no diabetes, nothing. With healthy eyes I would be in a very, very good condition, apart from now being too fat out of frustration. This was … the reason for the beginning of my spiritual quest. In my case extraordinary spiritual power is necessary for my healing. New retina cells must be produced and the retina in the left eye must be re-attached… Currently I try again 'cellevelhealing'. *They had amazing results. I already got 3 treatments, two more are scheduled, [but] till now no result, let us see.*"

The last sentence of this letter, underlined, already points to the Life-Medical 'diagnosis' that was arrived over seven months of correspondence with the patient. For though it begins with a claim that the healing method referred to by the patient had "amazing results", it concludes with a totally contradictory admission that "till now no result". The patient then adds "let us see" – but seems oddly *blind* to the contradiction, as if unwilling to face up to the fact or *see* that the method had not had the "amazing results" he wanted for himself.

I have italicised the word '*see*' both because of its relation to the patient's sight (which has since deteriorated by a further 10% in one eye) and also because of countless similar examples of statements made by the patient in the course of his correspondence with the Life Doctor – in all of which he appeared not to have understood or 'seen' what the Life Doctor had written to him – giving rise to the conclusion that he did not actually *want to see*. I should stress that the patient did not initially know about Life Doctoring or write to the Life Doctor as a *therapist* but rather as a spiritual teacher and *yogin* – someone who the patient believed could either heal him instantly or help him to develop extraordinary yogic powers with which to miraculously heal himself.

As a result, most of the patient's initial correspondence was *very narrowly focussed* on questions relating to detailed terminological and 'technical' aspects of yogic practice. Here again I emphasise the term *narrowly focused* – with its optical and visual connotations. Indeed, on many occasions the Life Doctor deliberately opted for *visual metaphors* in his correspondence with the patient in order to emphasise their significance for his sight problems and even pointing out to him that he had done so – by referring for example to *blindspots* in his thinking. Over the course of the correspondence however, what became ever more clear was the patient's fundamental unwillingness to *see* yoga and meditation as a method of attaining profound *insight* into himself and into his own medical condition – rather than as offering a mere method or set of theories and techniques for attaining miraculous powers of self-healing.

Below are just a few examples of language used by the patient in his emails which show instead how *fixated* his spiritual 'vision' was on transcending his body and on using spiritual powers and his 'third eye' to instantaneously and miraculously "burn away" his condition rather than gain any *insight* into it – let alone that of any other human beings:

"It must be possible to bring divine perfection to the physical plane."

"It must be possible to heal instantaneously by yogic powers."

"I clearly refer to what is called 'a miracle' by ordinary human beings."

"I want to be physically strong and healthy like a ferocious tiger, a mental genius and a spiritual giant with remarkable powers."

On the other hand, he admits that *"it was always a struggle for me to meditate"* and that *"to identify with another human being is for me quite terrifying ... my own weaknesses are enough."*

Though right from the start of correspondence with the patient, it was recommended that he read materials on Life Doctoring, and ask himself the sorts of question a Life Doctor would do, he did not initially do so. And even when the basic principles of Life Medicine were shared with him through correspondence, the patient – like many in search of spiritual 'healing' – had great difficulty in truly 'seeing', let alone heeding the basic idea that a specific illness might hold a specific meaning for the individual, that this meaning might itself be something worthy of *meditating* upon – and that in this way his illness might itself have a spiritual message for him and come to serve as his principal spiritual teacher and healer.

Indeed it seemed at times that this particular patient's 'reading' of the Life Doctor's letters was highly selective – as if he often did not even *optically register* those parts of them dealing with the nature and meaning of illness – let alone take any interest in the suggestion that a particular illness is always *chosen* by the individual for a well-intentioned reason and that its history must be viewed in the larger context of the patient's life story, life world and relationships.

On the contrary, it became ever more clear that this patient's vision of attaining healing powers over his illness *and* the very sight problems he sought to heal were both in fact *symptoms* – symptoms made particularly *visible* through his written correspondence – in which he continued to show little understanding or interest in any form of 'enlightenment' based on illuminating and meditative *in-sight*. And even without any experience of it he adopted a stereotypical negative viewpoint that any form of insight-based counselling was merely 'dredging the mud'.

Given that this was a patient, who, despite his serious sight problems simply 'did not want to see' the point of Life Doctoring, the Life Doctor felt that all he could do was to share with the patient precisely this Life-Medical insight – which itself had all to do *with* the patient's lacking interest in and capacity for deep 'in-sight' into himself and others.

Below I cite from two emails that constituted part of the climax of the Life Doctor's attempt to get the patient to 'see' the meaning of Life Medicine and the potential benefits of Life Doctoring, albeit taking care to do so in a way that respected the patient's relationship to him as 'spiritual teacher':

"All that you write confirms to me there may indeed be an important role that Life Doctoring can play in your life – though in a way very different from seeking a spiritual or biological 'miracle' cure of any sort. For I see your spiritual search for a miracle cure as more of a hindrance than a help.

The reason is that every healer you have been too, and every form of healing you have tried in order to find a cure for your eye condition is essentially a denial that it has any meaning. It seems that for you, as well as for the doctors and healers you have gone to, the only 'meaning' of your illness and what it can teach you seems to lie in finding a way to get rid of it.

But think of it this way: if your illness wants to be your most intimate and important spiritual teacher but all you want to learn from it is how to annihilate that illness – then you are looking for ways to annihilate your own teacher – in fact trying to kill it!

If and when you are ready to accept that this might be the most basic and important in-sight I can give you, then we can begin to consider ways and means in which, with my help – and through the reading and writing you are still (miraculously!) able to do – Life Medicine and Life Doctoring might bring you to a different and to a healing understanding of what your illness might be seeking to teach you.

From the point of view of Life Medicine 'the illness is the cure'. Life Doctoring is about finding out what the illness is attempting to cure in the patient!!!"

A short response to this message was then received from the patient in which he stated:

"... I really do not know what it is that I do not want to see. I will meditate that."

Since the Life Doctor's own email had already indicated to the patient what it was he did not want to see, a second e-mail was sent under the subject header 'What I see you as not seeing...' – once again making this as explicit as possible in the hope that this time the patient would 'see it'.

Your questions and vision have always been very <u>narrowly focussed</u> on 'techniques' of meditation. Throughout our correspondence however, I have tried to encourage an insight-based approach to your questions rather than a purely detached and technique-based one. I believe cultivating such an insight-based approach to life is also of central importance in relation to your eye problems.

You write that you "do not know what it is that I do not want to see".

So how about looking inside??!! And also listening inside and feeling inside.

That way you can come to your own answers – your own in-sights.

That is why I believe it terribly important that you learn to understand 'meditation' in a new way – not just as a set of techniques but as taking time to look inside yourself – for insights that can arise from feeling awareness.

Unless you learn to value deep personal and philosophical in-sights much more than you value yogic techniques and powers, and unless you learn to look inside yourself to feel for and find such insights, then I fear your eyes will just force you to do so.

For through increasing loss of 'out-sight' or even blindness you may eventually be unable to do anything <u>but</u> 'look inside' and also <u>listen</u> more deeply to yourself and others.

Put simply, through the decrease in your vision I believe <u>your eyes themselves</u> are telling you what you don't see – namely that despite all your knowledge and will power, without valuing and cultivating feeling in-sight, but instead continuing to narrow your thinking and spiritual vision either to detached intellectual and theoretical knowledge or to mastering yogic powers and *techniques to exercise in a detached way over your body, then your inner self or Atman will continue to narrow the vision of one or both of your bodily eyes through retinal detachment and eventually cut off your 'out-sight' completely. In other words, your illness – as your spiritual teacher – is saying that if you refuse to see inside you will lose your outer sight. It is therefore also urging you to put all your efforts into <u>seeing the difference</u> – perhaps for the first time in your life – between knowledge and wisdom, between your detached intellect and theoretical knowledge and deep feeling insight into yourself – and between manipulative techniques on the one hand and basic inner truths on the other. Using theoretical knowledge to attain power <u>over</u> your body from a detached ego or I are no substitute for your body's own inner knowing and powers of healing – and certainly no remedy for a detached retina in your eye – a clear symbol of your own detachment from yourself and others.*

The only substantive response to the message of these letters – and to an accompanying request for them to be incorporated into a case example in this book – was puzzlement that the author should wish to present a case study in which the patient had not been healed. This of course, simply re-affirmed the patient's misunderstanding of Life Medicine and Life Doctoring as an approach to medicine whose validity could only be proven by its effectiveness in healing the patient's illness – rather than offering potentially *life-transforming* and *healing understandings* of and insights into that illness. As for the idea that an illness might be there to *heal and transform the patient* – it was, again, simply not seen or registered on the mental *retina* of this patient – 'the man who did not want to see'.

On Life Doctoring

What is Life Doctoring?

LIFE DOCTORING is therapeutic counselling for serious or chronic illness. It is about 'treating the patient and not the illness' – by exploring links between illness and life – in particular the relation between the emergence of symptoms and significant life changes.

"It is changes that are chiefly responsible for disease." Hippocrates

What is a Life Doctor?

A Life Doctor is a psychotherapist trained in Life Medicine and able to provide Life Doctoring for symptoms of all sorts, both 'mental' and 'physical'.

A Life Doctor is not a conventionally trained biomedical doctor and is not qualified to prescribe any form of conventional medical treatment.

Yet a Life Doctor is not only a medically well-informed counsellor and consultant, but also possesses different types of medical knowledge and understanding of a sort that ordinary doctors do not receive in their training.

The Life Doctor will never seek to prevent a patient seeing or seeking advice from an ordinary doctor or medical specialist, but will instead explore the patient's experience of orthodox medical practice and practitioners and the meaning this experience holds for them.

The Life Doctor however, will ask questions of a sort very different to those put by ordinary doctors or specialist consultants – whose main role is to come to a biomedical 'diagnosis' of a patient's symptoms and to offer corresponding forms of treatment.

The Life Doctor will also advise the patient about the possible dangers and/or side effects of different forms of biomedical testing and treatment.

What Life Doctoring offers:

Opportunities for you to share your personal experience of illness and of medical services and treatments with a knowledgeable and informed counsellor independent of the medical profession.

Quality listening time – and a different type of listening – of a sort that doctors and consultants have no time for.

Healing of a sort that can only begin with being fully *heard* as an individual *human being* – not reduced to a 'case' of some hypothetical 'disease'.

Advice in making informed choices about medical tests and treatments, including their potential dangers and side-effects.

Help in revealing the true story of your illness – its biographical as well as 'medical' history – as well as its impact on your current life.

Awareness of possible relational dimensions of your illness – its connection to your personal, family and social relationships, past and present.

The chance to discover significant links between your illness on the one hand and significant changes and events in your past or present life on the other.

Ways to put you more in touch with your body and what it may be telling you – or seeking to tell others.

Greater trust in your body's own knowing as opposed to any body of medical beliefs.

Help in bringing to light the questions your illness may itself be there to make you ask yourself about your life.

Help in understanding and relating to your illness in ways free of the fears that diagnostic label s so often arouse.

New forms of healing based on meditating our bodies rather than medicating them.

Important knowledge, advice and support in preparing for consultations with doctors, consultants, surgeons or other health professionals.

Prevention from getting entrapped by standard medical or psychiatric procedures – being reduced to a mere 'case' of some clinically diagnosed disease.

Protection from being persuaded into accepting potentially dangerous, counter-productive or even life-threatening forms of orthodox bio-medical testing and treatment.

The Practice of Life Doctoring (1)

Life Doctoring is therapy for serious and chronic illness. Its focus however, is on the patient's felt or lived body and not just on the clinical body or the body seen merely as a complex biological machine. The Life Doctor understands the body not as a biological machine but as a living biological language of the human being and symptoms of illness as the 'speech' or expression of the patient's life situation, life world and life history as a whole. The practical starting point of Life Doctoring is therefore precisely the type of questions in my chapter on *What Most Doctors Don't Ask*. These relate to what was going on in the patient's life preceding the onset of symptoms, what they stop or hinder the patient from doing, the thoughts and feelings that accompany their symptoms and how they make the patient feel – that is to say, in what way they alter the patient's very sense of self – their body identity. At the same time, like any doctor, the Life Doctor must take a complete medical history of the patient – including all forms of testing and treatment they have undergone, what they have been led to believe about their condition and their experience of how they have been handled by doctors and other medical professionals.

The Life Doctor must also be capable of in-depth research and understanding of purely biological and biomedical understandings of the patient's condition. Like the General Practitioner, the Life Doctor is essentially a 'generalist' and not a specialist in these conditions. What distinguishes the Life Doctor however, is their capacity to 'read' even the most detailed biological and biomedical accounts of the nature and 'causes' of an illness in a very different way from that of a biomedical physician. For often the very language and terminology used in biological medicine itself, and the biological processes they are used to describe, can themselves be highly *symbolic*. This applies even to the very *names* given to certain conditions – for example the diagnostic term *lupus erythematosus* – meaning 'red wolf' and associated with dermatological symptoms such as red patches on the skin.

"Systemic lupus erythematosus ... often abbreviated to SLE or lupus, is a systemic autoimmune disease (or autoimmune connective tissue disease) that can affect any part of the body. As occurs in other autoimmune diseases, the immune system attacks the body's cells and tissue, resulting in inflammation and tissue damage. It is a Type III hypersensitivity reaction caused by antibody-immune complex formation. The course of the disease is unpredictable, with periods of illness (called *flares*) alternating with remissions. The disease occurs nine times more often in women than in men, especially in women in child-bearing years ages 15 to 35, and is also more common in those of non-European descent."

Wikipedia

Case Example 5

The patient in question first began to experience symptoms of lupus after coming off a treatment course of anti-depressants which lasted many years. The depression had followed the death of her grandmother, with whom she had a highly ambivalent relation. The symptoms of lupus had recently 'flared' again when it became a matter of financial importance to consider selling her mother's house – which she now occupied together with her partner but which the grandmother – a family matriarch – had insisted should always remain in the family.

As a woman, the patient felt responsible and sympathetic to the idea of maintaining a matriarchal line. On the other hand, she harboured deep feelings of anger at the way her mother had always been treated by the grandmother. These unexpressed feelings of anger and rage prevented her from, in any way, mourning the death of the grandmother and led instead to years of affect-less depression – the lack of affect being intensified by the anti-depressants themselves. Even after coming off them however, the patient's anger itself had never been given an opportunity to fully 'flare up'.

In consultations with the Life Doctor the patient gave a consistent impression of meek submissiveness – a strong parallel to her mother's submissive position in relation to the grandmother. At the same time the patient also experienced a sense of guilt at the idea of selling the house passed down by her grandmother. For to do so would be a betrayal, not just of the grandmother herself, but of the patient's own 'feminism', which had long found expression in an interest in Wiccan and other pagan forms of religiosity involving worship of the feminine aspect of divinity (which is sometimes called the 'great mother' – itself another term for 'grandmother').

The Life Doctor's analysis of the patient's illness in the context of her life history was that it was essentially rooted in a conflicted 'love-hate' relationship to her grandmother. On the one hand, she identified with what the grandmother symbolised for her (identification being an essential element of 'love') whilst on the other hand hating her for the way she had aggressively mistreated her own mother and reduced her to a state of passive servility. This is where the medical terminology itself revealed a new symbolic layer. For from the perspective of Life Medicine, auto-immune disorders – in which the body attacks itself – are an expression of guilt. The patient *punishes* themselves physiologically for feelings of guilt by directing the anger behind this guilt inwardly (through the body seeing its own cells as foreign or 'non-self') rather than this anger being consciously directed outwardly towards its true object – in this case the patient's grandmother.

"There are several explanations ventured for the term *lupus erythematosus*. *Lupus* is Latin for wolf, and *erythro* is derived from ερυθρός, Greek for 'red'. All explanations originate with the reddish, butterfly-shaped malar rash that the disease classically exhibits across the nose and cheeks.

1. In various accounts, some doctors thought the rash resembled the pattern of fur on a wolf's face.

2. In other accounts, doctors thought that the rash, which was often more severe in earlier centuries, created lesions that resembled wolf bites or scratches.

3. Another account claims that the term "lupus" did not come from Latin directly, but from the term for a French style of mask that women reportedly wore to conceal the rash on their faces. The mask is called a 'loup', French for 'wolf'."

Anger and rage are of course associated with the colour red – and for a biomedical diagnosis of *lupus erythematosus* (red wolf) the appearance of thick red patches or blisters on the skin is highly significant. So much for the 'red' in 'red wolf' but what about the wolf – itself an aggressive and predatory creature. The Life Doctor's interpretation of the patient's illness came to clearest expression through an intuitive link between the biomedical name and nature of her illness, her life history – and their common relation to the story of 'Little Red Riding Hood'. To the Life Doctor the patient appeared as 'Little Red Riding Hood'. The question was then – who 'ate' her grandmother? Clearly not a wolf, but perhaps someone who felt aggressive 'h-ate' for her i.e. a part of the patient herself. The patient's inability to mourn her grandmother's death might also therefore have been due to her feeling that her own suppressed feelings of hate were what killed her grandmother, thus compounding the patient's guilt. In a nutshell then, the patient developed symptoms of the illness known as 'red wolf' by virtue of never allowing herself to affirm, identify with and live out – what the wolf in the story symbolised – not just her blood-red anger towards the grandmother but the aggressive side of herself as a whole.

The key question for the Life Doctor then, was not how to 'treat' or 'cure' the lupus (it is regarded even in biomedicine as incurable) but rather an entirely different *type* of question. This was the question of what the illness was seeking to cure in the patient – in what way it was seeking to transform her? In the context of her particular history and the Red Riding Hood fable, it seems this question could be put more specifically: in what ways, besides 'flares' of her symptoms and bodily inflammations, did or did not the patient grant herself permission to consciously get 'inflamed' or 'flare up' with anger – and to fully feel, embody and show the true face of this anger? For this would allow herself to live out the 'red wolf' within her – rather than playing the role of 'little red riding hood' in relation to that wolf.

The personal significance of the fable for this patient lay in the way that the wolf symbolised *both* the aggressive side of
232

her grandmother and the patient's own feelings of anger toward her. In a sense it could be said that the patient, like her mother, had quite simply 'swallowed' her grandmother – not in a consciously predatory, hostile or aggressive way but by simply internalising or taking the grandmother inside herself – where she became the object of chronic or recurrent auto-immune attacks by her own body – which simply embodied the patient's dual and conflicted relation to the grandmother – both identifying with her as a part of herself and at the same time dis-identifying with her – leading the body to identify and attack her own cells as if they were 'foreign' or 'non-self' bodies.

The unconscious, internal and biologically routed attack on her grandmother no doubt further exacerbated the patient's chronic psychological guilt – thus creating a vicious cycle which maintained the symptoms of lupus – chronically recurrent symptoms.

The bodily symptoms themselves also corresponded to a specific state of consciousness characterised by a felt sense of weakness and therefore in themselves symbolised a type of recurrent submission *to* the grandmother – even whilst biologically symbolising an attempt to dis-identify from her on a cellular level – thus rendering her own cells subject to auto-immune 'attack'.

Yet, as mentioned, the patient came to the Life Doctor in a specific life situation in which her guilt – and the aggressive anger behind it – were exacerbated by the conflict she felt at perhaps having to sell her grandmother's house, this exacerbation leading to what biomedicine itself terms a 'flare' of the lupus. Biomedicine seeks causes for such flares in so-called 'environment al triggers' such as allergens, bacteria or viruses. Yet in this way the 'environment' in question is in no way connected with the patient's life world – their social and relational environment as a *human being* – but instead reduced to a possible source of infections or inflammations affecting the human body. Life Medicine, on the other hand, understands 'environmental triggers' as having *essentially* to do with particular events in the patient's social and relational environment – precisely because it is emotional triggers coming from this environment that may render an individual more *susceptible* to 'environmental triggers' in the purely biomedical sense.

Biomedical treatment of lupus symptoms takes the form of both anti-malarial and so-called 'anti-inflammatory' or 'immuno-suppressant' drugs. Both are an attempt to render the patient's body biologically *incapable* of expressing – through auto-immune responses and bodily inflammation – deeply buried and inflamed *feelings* which, in the absence of direct vocal, emotional or behavioural expression, will naturally seek a way of 'flaring up' and of literally 'coming to the surface' through *skin* inflammations. Yet if prevented from doing so by biomedical drugs, the danger is that the 'inflammation' will progressively begin to damage internal organs too – thus distracting the focus of both doctor and patient even further from the *basic question* of what the illness is there to 'cure' in the patient i.e. what understandings it is offering the patient and how it is seeking to change the patient in a way that would allow them to embody and express their dis-ease in a way other than through bodily illness and its symptoms.

Here again we come to the central question of Life Medicine, both in general and as exemplified in particular through so-called 'auto-immune' disorders – namely the potential role of the Life Doctor in acting as a midwife in helping patients feel and give birth to a new bodily *sense of self* or 'body identity' – as opposed to remaining stuck with an over-rigid or internally conflicted body identity that finds expression only biologically and through illness symptoms. In the specific case of the patient referred to here, she came to
234

recognise that the key to turning her illness into a cure lay in finding ways to overcome weak and submissive sides of her identity and instead to embody her anger and rage in ways that avoided the need for aggressive flares of her symptoms – flares which were also accompanied by periods of severe physical weakness. Here she was helped by some of the principal non-verbal methods of Life Doctoring explained and described in more detail in the following chapter on the Practice of Life Doctoring.

In this case the patient was asked to simply feel in her body and show the Life Doctor – silently and face to face – the true *face* of her feelings; both her un-mourned feelings of sadness but also her *anger* in relation to her grandmother (or to anyone). The exercise proved strongly cathartic for the patient in first surrendering to her sense of sadness and weakness and then feeling and showing the face of her anger. This was not a face marred by the red patch symptomatic of *lupus* but did indeed have qualities of aggressive fierceness of a *wolf-like* character – as opposed to the patient's previously *pale-faced* expression and submissive or compliant demeanour. The patient also understood the difference between allowing herself occasional emotional flares or verbal 'outbursts' of anger on the one hand, and, on the other hand using continued practice of the exercises she had been taught to silently *body* that anger through her facial expression and the look in her eyes – knowing from experience that in this way she could be coming to embody a new, less weak, sad or submissive sense of self, feeling it pervading her felt body and transforming her as a whole. It should be emphasised here that in dealing with long-term or chronic conditions, long-term practice of exercises introduced by the Life Doctor are of no less importance than the healing insights and understandings that Life Medicine offers.

The practice of Life Doctoring however, always begins with a search for the 'hidden story' behind a patient's illness in the form of what is called a 'pathobiography'. And indeed psychoanalysts such as Luis Chiozza have evolved a specific form of medical practice which they call 'the pathobiographical method'. This involves gathering a detailed biography of the patient which is then analysed by a team which includes not only psychoanalysts but also physicians and biomedical specialists. One important difference between Chiozza 's method and the practice of Life Doctoring however, lies in the fact that the latter does not rely on any form of elaborate psychoanalytic theory or esoteric terminology to 'interpret' the symbol ism of a patient's illness. Instead it attends purely and simply to what Freud called 'organ speech ', and in particular to four distinct ways in which this finds expression:

1. In the language of biomedicine itself – for example by re-linking the purely medical meaning of terms such as 'inflammation' or 'flare' to their use in describing emotional states ('flaring up' or 'feeling inflamed' with anger).

2. In the physiological symptoms, functions and processes described in the language of biomedicine (for example the language of immunology and of auto-immune disorders).

3. In the individual patient's lived experience of specific symptoms – as described in their own speech and as an expression of their lived or felt body.

4. Through the ways in which the specific life story and context of an individual patient's illness and its symptoms lends them a highly *individual* meaning.

In the past, and still in the work of Chiozza himself, psychoanalytic medicine has tended to seek 'standard' analyses of particular illnesses. This is not to say that there are no general understandings that can be drawn about the life meaning of particular organic disorders or dysfunctions – but this can be done only through Life Doctoring i.e. through exploration of highly *individual* cases of them. Life Medicine then, is not just a set of fixed general principles to be applied in and to particular 'cases' but is an expanding body of medical knowledge drawn from the very practice of these principles through 'Life Doctoring' – which serves also as a form of *on-going research* into the relation between language, life and illness.

The Practice of Life Doctoring (2)

As a practice, Life Doctoring is not simply a type of counselling or analytic 'talking cure'. That is because its principal focus is not on the causes and 'cures' but on the *meaning* of a specific illness and specific symptoms for the individual patient. Just as importantly however, as a form of therapy its principal 'instrument' is not just a new body of intellectual knowledge and insights but the Life Doctor's own lived body as a whole, their body of feeling awareness or 'soul'. It is only in this way that the Life Doctor can come to *directly* sense and resonate with the underlying *dis-ease* that pervades the patient's own soul and its body. Cultivating the capacity to sense the felt soul-inwardness of a patient's body takes us to a level much deeper than intellectual insight or emotional empathy alone. For the individual's lived body is essentially not a fleshly body of tissue and organs but a "body without organs" (Deleuze), the body of the patient's own *feeling awareness* of themselves, other people and the world around them. As such it is composed of particular tones, textures and tissues *of* feeling awareness. Like audible *vocal or musical tones* these silent feeling tones or tonalities of awareness have their own distinctive qualities such as tonal pitch and tone 'colour', brightness or darkness, warmth or coolness, lightness or heaviness, flatness or sharpness, softness or hardness, clarity or dullness, hollowness or resonance, harmony or dissonance. They are not just echoed in vocal and musical tones but also embodied in cellular, organic tone and muscular tone. Felt tonalities of awareness or feeling tones are what not only tone and colour our moods but also determine, in a quite literal sense, the 'sound-ness' of our health.

Particular 'elemental' *qualities* of feeling tone however – qualities such as fiery vitality, airy spaciousness, watery fluidity or earthly solidity may be more or less dominant or lacking. Thus, in the previous case example, the Life Doctor sensed a deep quality of warmth but a far lesser degree of both fieriness and solidity in the patient's overall feeling tone - an absence echoed also in the corresponding qualities of the patient's tone of voice. Part of the therapy also consisted of 'voice training' – teaching the patient to introduce a greater solidity, strength, amplitude and quality of fiery vitality to her voice tone. This was not done though any standard methods of 'voice coaching' but through first attuning her to particular qualities of her own inwardly heard speech – her 'inner voice' and its tones – and then imparting these tones of her inner voice with particular qualities of feeling tone, volume, fullness etc. – all *before* vocalising them audibly.

This particular method of Life Doctoring is one of many designed to *amplify* the patient's awareness of silent inner tones of feeling precisely *by* giving them outer expression – whether through the voice tones or silently, through their face and eyes. The basic methodological principle at the root of all these practices is the principle of 'Morphic Resonance', a term coined by Rupert Sheldrake but which Life Medicine understands in a very specific way - and that the Life Doctor applies through a very specific practice I term 'Morphic Resonation'. Both the principle of morphic resonance and the practice of morphic resonation are based on the understanding that by giving expressive outer form (*morphe*) to particular feeling tones (in particular through the voice, face and the look in our eyes) we both *amplify* and bring ourselves into greater *resonance* with these feeling tones – and thereby with our lived body as such.

Life Medicine understands the patient's visible 'physical' body as a *sensory image of their soul and its body*. Hence also, the patient's body language or 'body speech' (silent and vocal) is not only a fundamental dimension of what Freud called 'organ speech' but can also be used to give form to, amplify and *alter* a patient's sense of the felt mood or tone pervading their own feeling awareness and *its* body – their soul body or lived body:

"The outer shape of a person reflects his inner mood. Changing that shape can change his mood." David Boadella

Here 'shape' has the same meaning as *morphe* or 'form' in the term 'morphic resonation'. It can refer to anything from a particular posture, tilt of the head, or any feature, however fleeting of a person's facial expression and the look in their eyes.

"Consciousness in another's face. Look into someone else's face, and see the consciousness in it, and a particular shade of consciousness." Ludwig Wittgenstein

Perhaps *the* single most innovative and advanced method of Life Doctoring – and one that requires much training is practiced through extended, close-up eye contact with the patient. Here the Life Doctor uses the motility and expressiveness of his or her own face and eyes to seek for and precisely *mirror* particular features that he sees and senses in the patient's face and their eyes – features that no matter how subtle or fleeting can be seen and felt to give expression to the patient's innermost sense of 'dis-ease'.

Through this very precise *art* of facial and ocular mirroring the Life Doctor can:

1. *Attune* to particular tones and qualities of feeling in the patient by consciously observing and intentionally mirroring them back to the patient.

2. *Amplify* both their own and the patient's lived experience of these tones and qualities of feeling – thus bringing the patient into greater contact with them.

3. *Transform* the patient's experience of these tones and qualities of feeling, in particular by moving from a stage of mirroring the patient's 'emotional' feelings to mirroring these back purely *as* tones of feeling – comparable to purely musical tones and their sensuous qualities.

This three-stage method of Life Doctoring I call 'Transformative Resonance'.

In the previous case example, it was applied by the Life Doctor in roughly the following way:

1. By the Life Doctor sensing with their lived body as a whole and then mirroring back through the look in their own eyes and face in an expressively intensified way the surface look of resignation, surrender and 'sadness' seen in the patient's face and eyes.

2. By also sensing and mirroring back in intensified way glimpses of the weakly felt 'anger' latent within that sadness.

3. Sensing and mirroring this 'anger' back in a transformed way i.e. not merely as an 'emotional' feeling but as a purely *sensuous* feeling of power, strength and fiery vitality arising from the very core of the patient's lived body.

4. By imparting to the patient's lived body *as a whole* the Life Doctor's own bodily feeling awareness of this quality of fiery strength and vitality.

The recognition of the importance of the face and eyes in all forms of therapy is not new. And it must therefore play a central role in any form of therapy in which the therapist takes the client seriously as 'some-body' – not just a 'talking head'. Mirroring a patient's facial expression and the look in their eyes facilitates a process of mimesis which is central to sensing, attuning to and resonating with the patient's lived body as a whole.

"Without ... willingness to read the secret expression and to nurse it into life, any therapeutic encounter is gravely weakened."

"Facing is concerned with recognition, with how we see people, with the qualities of lumination that develop when people really face each other and with the forms of illumination that flash out of such contact. Insight develops in step with outlook.

If a person can let his inner self be seen by another, he begins to become recognisable to himself and can then look within, not in the sense of any sterile introspection, but in the sense of learning to love and accept who he is, and so recognise himself."
David Boadella, *Lifestreams*

Boadella also quotes an account of Wilhelm Reich's work with a patient who suddenly began "seeing the world with new eyes", the fear and hate having gone out of them. As a result he also saw his therapist differently. The process began with Reich noticing a new gleam in the patient's eyes, which...

" .... together with the shifting of the eyes and head, had brought up a new expression out of the depths of his eyes and being. It was a flirtatious, come-hither look, a sort of wink, with a raising of the eyelids, eyebrows and forehead and a moving of the eyeballs to one side, accompanied by a suggestive tilting of the head, in the same direction. As the therapist began to imitate this expression and the patient began to make better contact with it, the whole face participated in it, at first with a blushing shame-facedness, and then to the tune of a hearty laugh." (ibid)

Reich did not merely "face" or "confront" the patient with a *verbal* mirror or interpretation of what he had seen and felt in the face and eyes of the patient but used his own body to mirror it back directly – thus helping the patient to feel it more fully. As a result a "miracle" happens:

242

"Suddenly the patient was startled and opened his eyes wide with astonishment. While he was looking at the therapist the latter's face had suddenly become soft, and glowed with light...He saw the world differently, as a good and pleasurable place to be in and as a future place of 'heaven' and not the 'hell' it had been before." (ibid)

Bodily sensing and identification is involved even in the understanding of verbal and indeed philosophical thinking itself. Wittgenstein again:

"I begin to understand a philosophy by feeling my way into its existential manner, by reproducing the tone and accent of the philosopher."

The Life Doctor must be trained in many highly subtle and multi-faceted arts or 'yogas' of bodily sensing and resonance – all based on the principle of morphic resonance and allowing the practice of Transformative Resonance through 'morphic resonation'. This training begins with cultivating the Life Doctor's capacity to quite literally see into and experience a patient's eyes as 'windows of the soul' and, through looking into them, to use their own lived body as a whole to sense, resonate with and transform the particular "shade of consciousness" pervading the patient's own bodily feeling awareness of themselves.

It is in this way that the Life Doctor can also gain a tangible sense of those tones and qualities of feeling *not* fully embodied or expressed by the patient, but instead 'somatised' – given symbolic expression through their symptoms.

"Every feeling is an embodiment attuned in this or that way, a mood that bodies in this or that way." Martin Heidegger

What distinguishes Life Medicine and its therapeutic methods from those of psychoanalysis is that psychoanalytic theory understands illness symptoms only as symbolic 'somatisations' of feelings that the patient is not capable of articulating verbally. 'Somatisation', in other words, is understood solely as a failure to give expression to unconscious feeling in words – hence the emphasis of psychoanalysis on verbalisation and verbal interpretations of the symbolism of dreams and mental images.

In contrast, Life Doctoring understands 'somatisation' as a failure to find ways to consciously *embody* feelings through the patient's overall body language and body speech, which verbal language and speech is itself but one dimension of since it is with our bodies that we also utter words. In other words, it is not just through some lack of emotional illiteracy or 'alexithymia' as it is called, but also and above all through lacking a rich and expressive enough *body language* by which to 'speak' our feelings that what Freud called 'organ speech' is forced to take the form of illness symptoms or 'somatisation'.

It is not just that which we cannot express in words but above all that which we cannot expressively *embody* that we 'somatise'. Thus, referring back to our case example, it is not simply someone who cannot express or articulate a feeling of anger in words but principally someone who cannot simply *show* anger through their body speech – their posture, face and eyes - who is in greater danger of turning that anger inwards or somatising it. Indeed someone may well be capable of verbally reporting an emotion of anger (or any emotion) without or indeed instead of fully *feeling* it. For it is through expression in the 'shape' or form of their *body speech* that awareness of feelings (and of different tones *of* awareness or 'feeling tones') are not only given form but also *amplified* through resonance.

What is called 'emotional illiteracy' – to whatever degree it is evident and however important it is in itself – almost invariably *pales* in extent before the poverty of the average individual's body language and the limitations of their most basic 'alphabet' of postures, gestures, vocal tones, facial expressions and ways of communicating tones of feeling through the look in their eyes. This impoverishment of body speech and body language is in itself a form of generalised pathology – since it makes almost unavoidable the expression (*logos*) of a felt sense of dis-ease (*pathos*) through illness i.e. through 'pathological' bodily or behavioural symptom

.

Case Example 6

Patient: a 60 year old man teaching at a college and responsible also as a community elder for care and support of young people in difficulty.

Symptoms: heart arrhythmia, fainting spells, shortness of breath.

Biomedical diagnosis : atrial fibrillation (confirmed by ECG) and fibrosis of the lungs confirmed by X-ray – possibly connected through lack of sufficient oxygen and resultant shortness of breath.

Biomedical prognosis: possibility of early death (2-3 years) through progressive worsening of fibrosis in the lungs.

Medications prescribed: propranolol, badly tolerated because of side effects and replaced by sotalol – both intended to slow and regularise heart rate and reduce shortness of breath, Warfarin to reduce risk of stroke. Statins. Drugs to treat prostate enlargement.

Possible surgical interventions suggested:

- Heart surgery in the form of catheter ablation – used to destroy an area of the heart producing abnormal electrical circuits and resulting in disturbances of cardiac rhythm.

- Implantation of a pacemaker to regularise heartbeat.

Principle reasons for the patient arranging to see a Life Doctor:

- Concern about the prescribed medications and their actual or possible side effects.

- Dissatisfaction with what he experienced as a total lack of any expression of human warmth, empathy and interest on the part of the biomedical doctor s and consultants he had seen (not one of them even asked him about his feelings regarding the possibility of death within 3 years).

- Intrinsic interest in the approach to illness represented by Life Medicine and Life Doctoring.

Initial questions presented by the Life Doctor:

Questions regarding the patient's life history, work and current relationship.

Questions concerning the exact life time and location, life context and situation in which the symptoms first occurred, and how the patient felt and responded to them.

Questions regarding the frequency and exact situations and locations in which the symptoms of atrial fibrillation tend to re-occur.

Initial impressions and information gained by the Life Doctor:

The patient was felt as a human being with deep and natural warmth and empathy, humour and interest in others as well as in philosophical issues surrounding both methods of counselling and therapy and medicine itself.

Elements emphasised by the patient in sharing his life history:

- Early experiences of abandonment. His father abandoned his mother and himself when he was three years old. His mother however, who suffered from on-going withdrawal symptoms resulting from long-term dependency on psychoactive prescription drugs (benzodiazepine 'tranquilisers') also abandoned him in a different way. This took the form of lack of attention, empathy or sustained listening. Her resulting and constant inner restlessness, anxiety, depression and self-preoccupation expressed itself in extreme impatience if, as a child, the patient did not instantaneously reply to her questions. Not being given even a moment's time for reflection and authentic self-expression induced a severe childhood stutter in the patient, since overcome.

- Abandonment by the mother of his children, leaving him in the position of sole carer for three young children without any social or familial support whatsoever even from his brother or sister. This was reinforced by his sister-in-law, who refused to allow visits or even telephone calls with his brother. It was during this period that the patient's symptoms emerged.

- In contrast, the patient frequently emphasised how much he enjoyed the human contact with his students and how much appreciation they expressed for his warmth, humanity and overall bearing towards them – for example the way he did not 'talk down' to them as a teacher, but, as well as offering valuable teaching and insights, also related to them as human beings in their own right in an authentic and non-formal or role-bound way.

Initial links made by the Life Doctor between the patient's illness and his life circumstances:

- Life history of abandonment and the responses to it resulting from the patient's symptoms.

- Notably, it was only *through* an initial severe bout of his symptoms while living as an isolated single father that, despite his sister-in-law's prohibitions, he took the decision to phone his brother and actively seek support.

- The patient's decision to write to and consult with the Life Doctor was made not just in the context of his medical diagnosis and prognosis, but also his experience (through his mother and others) of the potentially damaging effects of prescription drugs and his sense of not being treated as a human being by medical professionals. Proactively contacting the Life Doctor thus constituted a way in which the patient's *illness itself* led him to enact a healthy part of himself – one that refused to surrender to many life experiences of relational isolation and abandonment.

Other felt impressions from the initial consultation:

- The Life Doctor observed that at no point in the initial consultation did the patient say how his initial account of his illness and life, together with his current medical diagnosis and prognosis left him feeling or thinking (a question which no one, even his current partner, had at any time asked him). Instead the 'patient' simply took great pleasure and interest in the opportunity the consultation provided for warm, informal but also patient and therefore insight-generating communication provided by the Life Doctor himself – both as a human being and as a man of similar age with whom he shared common life values, understandings and even experiences.

- On the other hand, the Life Doctor felt, through the patient's downcast gaze and generally lowered lids, a bodily sense of something like an underlying mood of resignation behind the patient's otherwise animated, open and interest-full vocal communication. The mood of resignation seemed in contrast to the proactive and healthy steps taken by the patient in response to his experiences of abandonment that his symptoms had led him to enact – leading ultimately to the pleasure and interest he took in the Life-Doctoring consultation itself and his interest in having further sessions. At the same time, the Life Doctor observed that the patient was taking more of an interest in the consultation itself than in his own feelings about his illness. Together with the sensed mood of resignation, the Life Doctor became even more curious about what the essential existential or life 'dis-ease' of the patient might be, particularly since the patient had also reported an acute episode of his symptoms in which he felt he might be dying – but also felt quite happy to let go and resign himself to death – therefore in effect abandoning himself.

Between life and death – the patient's essential life dilemma:

Knowing something of the circumstances surrounding the emergence of the patient's symptoms – and knowing also that despite the fibrosis of his lungs and occasional shortness of breath walking up steep inclines, the patient was still able to take mile-long walks without any difficulty – the Life Doctor returned in the second session to the patient's symptoms of atrial fibrillation and asked the patient how frequently and in what particular circumstances he tended to experience them. The answer was quickly forthcoming and revealing – whenever he was at home with his current partner, towards whom he had long felt a loss of sexual attraction, who did not share any of his interests, with whom he could not discuss his work as a teacher or any deeper philosophical and life questions. Indeed it was his partner herself who – although the patient described her as very "loving and caring" – made clear that she felt abandoned by him merely by his reading a book in her presence. Lacking all forms of physical contact and sexual fulfilment from the patient led to a progressive increase in the weight gain that had first diminished his sexual desire for her since they met. However she was also limited in her willingness and capacity to openly discuss their physical relationship. This was made worse by personal and cross-cultural differences which made even attempts at mutual discussion of the future of their relationship very difficult.

Placed in the context of the patient's radically different experience of his world of work, the picture that emerged was one of the patient inhabiting two entirely separate and contrasting life worlds. One world was the spacious, enlivening, emotionally heartening, intellectually inspiring and also libidinally restorative (if not fulfilling) world of his close, authentic and heartfelt relationships with his students and co-teachers. This was a world in which he was able to embody his deepest values and abilities as a human being, share his greatest interests and at least feel if not fulfil strong sexual desires. The other world was the narrow, enclosed and stifling world of his sexually and communicatively unsatisfying home life and relationship with his partner. For this, in contrast, was a world he experienced each day as disheartening and deadening – in contrast to the enheartening and enlivening relational world of his work and students in which he also felt 'room to breathe'. It became clear to the Life Doctor that the bodily mood of resignation he had sensed in the patient had to do with the way the patient had resigned himself to living in these two contrasting worlds – one enlivening and enheartening, the other disheartening and deadening – leaving him with a life quite literally led 'between life and death'. The Life Doctor shared with the patient the direct parallels he saw between this, the essential 'dis-ease' of the patient, and his potentially life-threatening or life-shortening heart and lung symptoms and the 'disease' or 'disorders' by which they were biomedically labelled.

The patient's response to the life picture of his illness:

In the third session, the patient, when questioned, reported how much he had reflected on, understood and agreed with the 'life picture' of his illness offered by the Life Doctor at the end of the second session and how he also saw the clear relationship it revealed between his lung and heart condition and his current life situation. In this session too however, it also became clear to both doctor and patient that, in the context of his life picture of his illness, the biggest threat to the patient's health and life lay not in any biomedically labelled condition or prognosis but rather in resigning himself to a life led 'between life and death', i.e. between two life worlds, the one alive and the other dead. The Life Doctor suggested that the alternative to resignation or self-abandonment in this limbo state lay in understanding the lived dis-ease and its bodily symptoms as the expression and embodiment of a fundamental life dilemma – one which demanded careful consideration and perhaps new and courageous life decisions from him, not least with regards to his relationship to and sexual life with his current life partner – with whom it became clear again that he was extremely 'ill-at-ease'.

In this context the Life Doctor became aware, following this session, of a particular paradox of the patient's life dilemma and the potential life decisions it demanded from him – namely that were he to leave his relationship with his partner or pursue new relationships whilst staying within it, he himself would become the abandoner rather than the abandoned. On the other hand, it was already evident that he had for a long time inwardly been afraid of or abandoned all attempts to rescue or redeem the relationship, as had his partner herself – leaving it in a state of routinized, uncommunicative and death-like limbo, one in which they inhabited separate worlds even whilst living together.

It was agreed that future sessions would concentrate on the life dilemmas and decisions faced by the patient, together with (1) on-going monitoring of when, in what situations, to what degree and how often his symptoms occurred and (2) continued discussion of whether – or which – of the several different prescription drugs he was taking were necessary. Questions of the role and potential influence on health exerted by different beliefs about death – and the existence or not of an afterlife – were also placed on the agenda for further exploration.

Observation of the patient's mood and body language:

Last but not least, the Life Doctor felt a need to address what he felt as the patient's underlying mood of resignation in the face of his life circumstances and dilemmas. This was expressed very strongly in the patient's body language – in particular the tilt of his head and body, the look in his eyes and his facial expression as a whole. The Life Doctor observed that the patient tended almost invariably to tilt his head down to one side and towards his left shoulder. This was accompanied by a type of worried frown which drew his eyelids together almost completely – as if squinting in the face of a bright light – making eye contact with others impossible.

It was as if the patient had over the years got stuck in a habit of never fully 'holding his head high' rather than leaning it down to one side – and found it now extremely difficult to do so. His 'downcast gaze', in other words, had effectively become part of his body identity, as had his tendency not to open his eyes fully so that he could not 'look people straight in the eye.

The Life Doctor responded to this by feeding back his observations of the patient's body language, mirroring them and explaining to him the principle that: *"The outer shape of a person reflects his inner mood"* (Boadella) and that *"Changing that shape can change his mood."*. Noting how even in close up eye contact with the patient – and despite attempts to straighten his head and neck – the patient still invariably held his head slightly tilted to one side, the Life Doctor gave the patient inter-session 'body homework'. This took the form of suggesting that he attempt to keep his head perfectly balanced and upright for an entire day or week – and to then see and feel how 'changing his shape' in this way and also looking people 'straight in the eye' might affect his bodily sense of self and alter both his mood of resignation and resigned mode of relating. For his current posture both embodied and reinforced these – not just in his relation to his partner but also his supervising manager.

Progression and Outcomes of the Life Doctoring Sessions:

The possibility of a less resigned and more proactive mode of relating – both verbally and bodily – was heeded by the patient with good results – initially however only in the context of his relationship to his supervisor, which he approached in a new, courageous and effective way.

Though he also made attempts to move closer to his partner, these were clearly not successful, and yet they gave further insight into his heart symptoms. For on further questioning he reported that his symptoms of atrial fibrillation started or became particularly acute not just in the presence of his partner but *specifically* on occasions when she indicated a desire for sex. The patient described how on such occasions he experienced strong inner feelings of guilt at not being able to *reciprocate* in any way the love and care he felt he received from her. Rather than openly and proactively sharing these feelings of guilt with her – which would itself have at least been a token of his reciprocal care for her – he would simply say he was "not in the mood ", hiding both his feelings and the episodes of atrial fibrillation that accompanied them. And though the patient took on board a suggestion to make time to honestly share his feelings with his partner – and his reasons for not wanting sex – he found this extremely difficult to do. He even found it impossible to offer his partner any form of affectionate non-sexual contact such as a hug. Recognising that in this way he was effectively 'abandoning' his partner, The Life Doctor suggested that this might be a way of acting out his own history of abandonment by others as well as being part of his general and long-term inability to experience intimate connection with women except through sexual arousal and intercourse.

With regards to the patient's other symptom – shortness of breath – its initial diagnosis and prognosis through X-ray scans as a specific form of fibrosis of the lungs, one which might progressively worsen and even shorten his remaining life span to two years, was brought into question. For when the patient met his medical consultant again and asked why a decision had been taken *not* to conduct any further scans but instead to just regularly monitor the patient's lung function capacity, the consultant effectively admitted that the initial scan was not conclusive.

As a result, the patient reported having no more worries at all about having a potentially terminal illness – since it was the seemingly premature *medical diagnosis and prognosis* itself that had really 'taken his breath away' – causing more anxiety than his shortness of breath itself. And in the course of his sessions with the Life Doctor these had become and remained so mild as to be hardly even abnormal. The patient instead reported going on long walks again – for him both a major source of pleasure in life and also his means, besides teaching, of enjoying a sense of friendship and non-sexual bonding and connection with others.

This is not to imply that the sessions of Life Doctoring constituted, in and of themselves, a 'cure' for the patient's illnesses, but rather an opportunity to let them serve as a cure for the patient – firstly by showing how they expressed important aspects and dilemmas connected with past and current life and relationships, and also by urging him to find a new body identity – one in which a basic mood of resignation to life could be transformed, quite literally, by learning to 'hold his head high' and 'look people firmly in the eye'.

Death by Prognosis and the 'Nocebo Effect' – a postscript to Case Example 6

More than *two years after* my work with the patient described in Case Example 6 – whose initial reason for coming to me was the fear evoked in him by having been told that given the condition of his lungs he had *only two years of life left* - I was most surprised to hear from him again by e-mail saying that he had *once again* been given a dire and dread-inducing medical prognosis – this time being told he had only *one year* left. The prognosis was initially given solely on the basis of a poor result from a lung function test - though, I as immediately suspected - but only much later admitted to him - this result could not in fact be regarded as evidence of anything, since it which was conducted shortly after he had a temporary chest infection. I should add here that the chest infection itself arose just after he had, once again, managed (and that in cold and damp winter weather) to take a series of *12-16 mile walks* with his friends on the Pennine Way – not exactly evidence of a man whose lungs are about to give in, and that despite his lung fibrosis.

I was very shocked to hear this news – knowing that according to his first prognosis he should have *already* been dead by now, and that it had taken only a couple of sessions in my work with him to lift the fears it had aroused in him. Indeed it seemed to me almost as if his physicians wanted him to die just in order to once again try and prove a flawed 'scientific' prognosis. Knowing also how *deeply depressed* he was at having long since lost the teaching job that was his principal source of meaning and enjoyment in life – as well as his sole source of income – and that he had almost no chance of getting another job, I offered him free consultations – both by phone, at home in my practice and through correspondence. In the course of these I learned that his fears of dying had, this time, been even further intensified by being referred to a specialist palliative care nurse, offered counselling for terminal illness and advice on writing a Will – even to the extent of being asked whether he had a pet that he might want included in it.

My shock turned into outrage however, when I learned, furthermore, that he had attended a meeting of mutual support group for patients with the same medical condition, and that at this meeting a hospital pharmacist had addressed the group in a clear attempt to persuade them to act as guinea pigs for a new and highly expensive drug (£30,000 per patient) that might extend their lives by a few months, yet doing so even *whilst admitting* that this very same drug had been "poorly trialled" and had side effects such as nausea, loss of appetite and liver toxicity that could significantly affect patients' quality of life.

I used my renewed sessions with this patient to conduct a 'breath test' of my own with him and also to share two important facts and research with him that he might not know of. The test I conducted was simply to feel the strength of his abdominal muscles by getting him to attempt to expand his abdomen against the pressure of my hand. The conclusion I shared with him was that a big question for me was not *how well or badly* he was capable of breathing (for despite his regular miles-long walking he did report occasional occasional experiences of shortness of breath) but *how he breathed.* That was because the result of my own test shocked me – for in all my years I had never encountered a client, student or patient with such totally flaccid abdominal muscles – or someone so wholly incapable of using these muscles – and not just his chest muscles – to breathe more fully and deeply (something I advise or train all my patients to do).

One of the important facts I shared with him was that for many years now (and although this came about principally as a result of litigation fears among United States physicians) even doctors in the U.K. National Health Service had been brainwashed to now consider it more 'ethical' to give their patients a *worst-case figure* when it came to their life expectancy. This new, supposedly more 'ethical' stance was confirmed by my patient's own wife when she questioned the doctors working at the medical clinic at which she was employed.

I also shared my research into what is called the 'nocebo effect' in contrast to the 'placebo effect': a placebo being a totally inert drug that appears to work simply because the patient is led to *believe and expect it will*, and a 'nocebo' being one that has harmful effects for the same reason – its effects on the patient's beliefs and expectations.

"The term *nocebo* (Latin *nocēbō*, "I shall harm", from *noceō*, "I harm") was chosen by Walter Kennedy, in 1961, to denote the counterpart of one of the more recent applications of the term *placebo* (Latin *placēbō*, "I shall please", from *placeō*, "I please"); namely, that of a placebo being a drug that produced a beneficial, healthy, pleasant, or desirable consequence in a subject, as a direct result of that subject's beliefs and expectations." Wikipedia

The concept of placebo and nocebo effects however, has been extended by medical anthropologists to embrace *any type* of medical procedure or even any type of behaviour of communication of physicians that effects a patient's beliefs and expectations. Thus the most effective doctors tend to be those who – in themselves and through their own way of relating to their patients, have a 'placebo effect' on then patients – for example by giving those patients both empathy and positive reassurance. In contrast it was all too clear that my own Life Doctoring patient was suffering from a strong and deeply troubling 'nocebo effect', one stemming not just from the pessimistic prognosis he had been given but the multiple bureaucratic procedures and referrals that followed it, in which a veritable army or 'task force' of drug companies, pharmacists, consultants, nurses and counsellors was targeted at him in a way that could only intensify his fears and negative expectations.

The concept of a nocebo effect has also been used to explain the phenomenon of 'voodoo death' – people dying as a result of a firm belief in the fatal powers of a witchdoctor's spells, curses or rituals, such as 'bone pointing' or giving someone the 'evil eye'. The modern definition is broader:

"*Voodoo death*, a term coined by Walter Cannon in 1942 also known as *psychogenic death* or *psychosomatic death,* is the phenomenon of sudden death as brought about by a strong emotional shock, such as fear. The anomaly is recognized as "psychosomatic" in that death is caused by an emotional response – often fear – to some suggested outside force. Voodoo death is particularly noted in native societies, and concentration or prisoner of war camps, but the condition is not specific to any culture or death.

Another scientist—Clifton K. Meador, MD—in 1992 discussed the case of a man diagnosed with cancer who, along with his physicians and family, believed he was dying of cancer. In the autopsy after his death, however, the doctors discovered that his cancer was not at all the cause of his death. Meador deduces that the man's belief in his imminent death was the cause of his death itself." Wiki

A third point was made by an associate of mine, himself a practicing doctor, who reminded my patient that the medical profession comes to clinical judgements, decisions – and prognoses – on the basis of patient 'clusters' (i.e. statistics) rather than by assessing patients as individuals.

Together it seemed that my patient was initially much encouraged by our talks and correspondence, writing "that I cannot thank you enough for your approach, resources and commitment, it has given me a different perspective..." and "...has really helped me to view the disease differently and abate the panic attacks..." He wrote also that "My major learning lesson has been that when we are vulnerable and passive, how much power we give up..." and of his failure to meet any professional he had spoken to who had heard of the 'nocebo effect' – let alone to take any interest in it or even give it a moment's thought.

Yet given the basic mood of morbid resignation towards life that had come to the fore in our first round of sessions, as well as the continued and deepening depression associated with his joblessness, general loss of meaning in life – and the fear occasioned by his 'new' prognosis – I was both immensely saddened and the same time not entirely surprised to learn, after just a two-month or so interval in our communication, that my patient had unexpectedly and quickly died. He did so in hospital following a recurrence of his chest infection after another round of what he still enjoyed most – walking. Yet it was his death that prompted me to write this chapter on 'Death by Prognosis and the Nocebo Effect', and it is to him – a most likeable, humble and gentle man, and one full of human warmth and kindness – that I dedicate it.

What can I do if I am a Biomedical Doctor?

Study more of the literature on Phenomenological, Existential and Psychoanalytic Medicine (See the list of 'Further Reading'.)

If you are in private practice, consider extending at least your initial consultations with each patient to up to an hour – to allow time to gather more information about their lives, life world and life history.

If you are working as a GP in the public health system:

Recognise and talk with your colleagues about the *counter-productivity* of short 7 or 10 minute consultations and emphasise instead the potential of longer consultations to actually *reduce* the workload of doctors – as well as deepening and enriching doctor-patient communication.

Less medical testing and more *talking* with your patients!

Ask more questions about the patient's life and not just the symptoms they present with.

In particular, take opportunities to ask questions of the sort listed in the section of this book called 'What Most Doctors Don't Ask'.

For even within a very time-limited consultation it is possible to gather at least some information on the life context of a patient's symptoms by opening a consultation with a friendly general question such as 'How are things going?' – giving time for the patient to offer more than just a superficial answer.

When a patient reports symptoms, ask 'Had anything been troubling you before the symptoms started?'

Allow yourself to reflect on and share with the patient any possible symbolic or metaphorical dimension to a patient's symptoms, relating to their current life problems and circumstances.

Example: itching or sensitive skin :

"Anything you've been itching to do?" "Anything you've been feeling particularly sensitive to recently?"

Example: stomach, digestive or bowel symptoms:

"Anything you've found hard to stomach/digest/get out of your system recently?"

Ask for and make notes of *dates* – not just the patient's date of birth but the birth and/or death dates of relatives, siblings or spouses. You can do this in the course of asking about diseases in the family such as diabetes, cancer or heart disease.

Be aware of the *timing* of appointments made by patients – these may coincide with the timing of significant events such as births and deaths of people whom the patient identifies or feels a strong connection with.

Be aware that *genetic* explanations of illness may *disguise something completely different* – a strong psychological feeling towards and/or identification with a member of the patient's family. The fact that illnesses are transmitted across generations does not mean that the mode of transmission is principally genetic.

Always find a way to ask the patient what's been going on in their mind in relation to their symptoms, for example the question:

"What sort of thoughts and feelings tend to accompany your symptoms and what thoughts do you tend to have about them?"

Menstruation, Migraine and Meaning –
A Short Lesson in 'Life Doctoring'

The following case offers a further example for biomedical doctors, emphasising the importance of (1) asking the patient *different type of questions* to those they might normally ask a patient (2) being alert to *symbolic* dimensions of a patient's symptoms and (3) seeing symbolic dimensions also to their own medical knowledge of a particular condition and its physiology (both in its typical and atypical manifestations in a given patient).

The aim is to show how taking this Life Medical approach can prove far more effective than simply approaching this condition in a standard way, e.g. by prescribing medications without consideration of *either* the life-context in which a patient's symptoms or condition emerged, its life meaning for the patient and the individual significance of both its typical and/or atypical aspects.

Case Example 7

The patient: a married woman in her late thirties who suffered from migraine for almost twenty years, at first irregular and non-menstrual related and then later becoming regular and menstrually related.

Questions to the patient:

When did the symptoms first occur?

The patient experienced her first, non-menstrual migraine during a stay at home from university during the summer holidays.

What were the most important life encounters, events, experiences or dilemmas preceding the onset of symptoms?

In this period she was effectively given the responsibility of 'head' of the family by her parents – having to both sort out family affairs and also take care of an elderly relative who she found quite repugnant.

Was there any sort of underlying mood accompanying the symptoms?

Yes, one of general negativity toward the tasks with which she was burdened but also guilt about her own negative feelings.

What did the symptoms force the patient to do, stop her doing or allow her to do?

The first strong migraine made it impossible for the patient to perform the tasks relegated to her by her parents. They forced her to spend days in a darkened room. In this way they also allowed her to take 'time out' from her tasks and give time to herself.

At what times do the symptoms tend to recur, intensify or diminish?

The patient's migraines had continued to recur irregularly for some years after the initial episode. Sometime after she embarked on her chosen career as a university lecturer, she got together with the partner she later married. The couple decided against having children because neither felt a need or wish to have a family. It was around this time that her migraines first began to recur regularly each month, before the onset of menstruation.

What did the patient do in response to her symptoms?

Taking medications in order to alleviate her symptoms sufficiently to able to 'function' in her work most of the time.

How did the symptoms, and the thoughts and feelings around them, affect the patient's life, work and relationships?

At first the patient's main aim was to use medication in order to not to let her migraines affect her work, which was an important medium of self-actualisation for her. As for her relationship however, though her husband had shared her choice to not have children, with the help of her psychotherapist the patient realised that she harboured some resentment about his seeming emotional indifference to the decision. After being encouraged by the therapist to feel her own feelings about her decision more deeply in her body – and to discuss the decision not to have children once again with her husband – the issue 'came to a head'. The patient was surprised to find that both she and her husband harboured feelings of sadness and loss at not having a family and that he was prepared to rethink should she change her mind. This removed her resentment toward what she had thought of as her husband's indifference and brought her closer together with him – whilst at the same time leaving her free to re-affirm her decision to stay childless. In the context of her long-term relationship, this did now *constitute* a concrete life decision in the true sense i.e. a definite choice between two available options.

What beliefs does the patient hold about their symptoms and the right way to respond to them?

The patient initially appeared to accept the standard socio-cultural beliefs made use of in the advertising propaganda put out by the pharmaceutical industry – beliefs which many doctors themselves are complicit in following. A principle belief is that with the help of the right 'off the counter' or prescription pill, patch, tampon, cream or pharmaceutical concoction there is never a need to not go sprightly and cheerfully out of the house and into the world and to stay economically active – whether you suffer from backaches, joint pains, headaches or even cyclical pre-menstrual symptoms. Indeed this applies particularly to menstruating women, who are given a graphic message through advertising that there is no need to not feel full of energy and unencumbered by the monthly 'curse'. Yet for a woman who is aware of her bodily and emotional needs, menstruation is a time to feel her body more fully and in this way also 'come back to herself', listen inwardly to her body and either grieve or rejoice that no child is on the way.

The menstrual cycle of course, follows the lunar cycle i.e. a healthy and natural cycle that all living beings are influenced by: a cycle of waxing and waning. This is one of many natural cycles – the cycle of expansion and contracting that can even be observed in the amoeba, the natural cycle of waking and sleeping, and a no less natural cycle of moving out into the world on the one hand, and withdrawing into one's self and body on the other.

Without phases of contraction no child would be born naturally. And without 'coming back to' or 'going down into' ourselves and our bodies we cannot feel ourselves or our bodies fully – and thus go out into the world and relate to others out of a fully re-embodied and authentic sense of self.

Current Westernised societies with their 24/7 culture however, no longer adhere to these cycles or natural rhythms and instead impose a constant 'forward' and 'out-going' movement as a normative way of living – negating the value of introspection, contraction or withdrawal from the world as unwelcome or even unhealthy and pathological conditions. That is why it is not surprising that both minor ailments such as headaches, colds and flues or even highly painful or discomforting symptoms or illnesses are so often needed as a 'cure' for what is effectively a *pathological* cultural norm – being the only socially acceptable way for individuals to break free of it – even if only by forcing individuals to take time out in which there is nothing to do but feel their bodies and thereby their own selves more fully – to *give time* to them.

Is there any positive and healthy side to the different mood and sense of self accompanying a patient's bodily symptoms – or to what their symptoms force or allow them permission to do – or not to do?

Are there any other ways in which the patient could give expression in their life to this positive and healthy side of their symptoms – without needing those symptoms as a spur to do so?

With the help of her psychotherapist – acting in the role of 'Life Doctor' – the patient herself quickly realised that she had deprived herself all her life of the benefits of a natural and healthy cycle of expansion and contraction. This was a breakthrough for the patient. It allowed her to recognise that the migraines – particularly when *not* medicated – forced her to slow down, to spend time with herself without working, reading, talking or distracting herself in other ways. She wondered whether this was what her body was trying to cure her of through her 'illness' and decided to see what happened if she started using this cure independently of the illness itself – for example by pacing herself more, allowing herself more time to not 'do' and just be, taking breaks instead of hurrying from one task to the other etc. So even though she continued to work very hard she no longer allowed the needs of work to dictate the natural rhythm of her day – and of her body – but began following her own. Even when she had to work 14-hour days she still made time to intersperse tasks with short breaks during which she allowed herself to be more consciously aware of her body and how she was feeling. About 3 weeks after changing her daily habits in this way – and doing so without feeling *guilty* for no longer following culturally imposed norms – she experienced her first migraine -free onset of menstruation in 15 years. Through her illness and the insights that also 'came to a head' through it, she hasn't had a migraine since – not because it was medically 'cured' but because she allowed the illness itself to help her 'cure' and overcome *unhealthy beliefs and an unhealthy way of living.*

What symbolic dimensions can be seen in the patient's symptoms and their history and what light do they shed on both menstrually and non-menstrually related migraine?

Both the symptoms of menstruation and those of migraine ask people to take 'time out' from their regular routines – or rather to take 'time in' – time to go into themselves, just be with and feel themselves more fully from within. The typical symptoms of migraine – painful headache, nausea, feeling sick and vomiting, sensitivity to light and noise can be seen as having two principal symbolic dimensions. One is the service they perform in bringing the effects of a culturally normative but essentially unnatural and unhealthy way of living 'to a head' – through painful headaches. The other symbolic dimension has to do with how sufferers respond to migraine attacks, which is often by shutting themselves off in a darkened room – as if recreating a *womb* for themselves shielded from light and sound.

Herein lies a symbolic clue, not only to the frequency of so-called 'menstrual migraine' in women, but also to the unmet needs of male sufferers. In the specific context of the patient referred to, it is symbolically interesting to note also that hers was a profession – university lecturer – focussed on use of the head. And in an age in which sedentary 'service' professions

268

and mental work dominates over farming or different forms of manual work, there is a far greater tendency for individuals to lose touch with their bodies – and in particular with the so-called 'gut brain' as opposed to the 'head brain '. For this, like the uterus, is located in the abdomen – which contains more nerve cells than the brain. Finally it is to be noted again that the patient's first episode of migraine, albeit non-menstrual, occurred at a time when, though supposedly on holiday, her time was filled with tasks that effectively demanded that she take on the role of *parent* in relation to her own parents. In this context, her migraine can be seen as serving an important and healthy balancing role by making her withdraw to a darkened room – thus allowing and encouraging her to both avoid and recover from the parental tasks placed on her by placing herself back in the position of a baby in a protective womb.

Though it is a not an uncommon condition, medical literature and practice never attempt to see any symbolic connection between 'menstrual' or 'menstrually related' migraine on the one hand, and a women's relation to both her periods and to having or not having children. This is of no small significance in a time and a culture where women are under greater pressure than ever either to manage the highly demanding and stressful role of 'working mother' or else to put the interests of their careers and employers ahead of motherhood. Of symbolic note here is also the fact that the use of standard hormonal contraceptives to avoid pregnancy are known to worsen the symptoms of menstrual migraine and are specifically contra-indicated for women over thirty five i.e. precisely those women reaching a critical life phase in terms of deciding whether to stay childless or not.

Philosophical Postscript
– Touch and the Essence of Bodyhood

"The tactile realm of perception is the same thing as the body."
Samuel Avery

So far in this book I have used terms such as 'lived body', 'felt body' or 'body of feeling awareness' to present another understanding of what we call 'the body' or 'a body'. I have also argued that the 'body of our feeling awareness' as a whole – our 'soul' – embraces the entire field or space of experiencing that we perceive as the 'world' around us. Here I wish to go a little further in exploring the single word 'body'.

To most people, of course, this word has a self-evident meaning which is rarely questioned. They see the human body, like any other 'body', as a bounded 'material' object in space. I stress the word 'see', for it hints at the way in which the dimension of visual experiencing has come to dominate both our perception and conception of the body and of bodies, i.e. of 'bodyhood' as such, leading us also to think of bodies as 'material' objects 'in' space.

In reality however, nobody ('no-body') can see, hear or even touch 'matter'. For what we call 'matter' is actually a purely *abstract concept* to which there corresponds no 'objective' reality we can directly experience or prove the existence of. Instead, what we think of as properties of 'matter' are simply qualities of *subjective* experiencing – in particular those qualities of *tactile* experiencing such as hardness or softness, weight and density, roughness or smoothness etc. In other words, it is only because something that we actually see in space is also sensed as something that can be *potentially* felt in a tactile way that we come to think of it *as* a 'material' body.

'Space' itself however, is no objective 'physical' dimension but rather the principal dimension of subjective visual *experiencing*. So again, what we 'see' in it is also only what we can also potentially feel or touch. Indeed we could go so far as to say that *visual* experiencing of and in 'space' is itself a sensory and spatial interpretation of *tactile experiencing* in all its dimensions, actual and potential - which include hearing, taste and even smell. For hearing is vibration that *touches* us - and gives us a sign of something that can potentially be touched. Similarly, smell gives us a sign of something that can potentially be tasted - taste itself being a form of touch. That is why a dog's experience of space is shaped as much - if not more - by their acute sense of hearing and smell than by sight alone.

As human beings, whilst we can see a plant or even a single-celled organism under a microscope – neither the cell nor the plant can either see, hear or even smell. What the plant senses, it senses only in a directly tactile way – whether as a breeze, insect or chemical on its surface. What a single cell experiences – even a cell of our own 'body' and its multiple 'sense organs' (a retinal cell for example) it experiences through touch and feeling awareness alone. It is only through the sense of sight that has been developed by 'multicellular organisms' that they come to interpret their tactile experience in a visual and spatial way – or that human beings in particular come to perceive and conceive 'cells' themselves (and the tissues, organs and bodies composed of them) principally as visual and 'material' objects – rather than *feeling* them subjectively in the tactile way that they feel themselves.

Yet given the fundamentally tactile nature of cellular experiencing it is no surprise that both touch and herbal remedies are amongst the oldest forms of healing – affecting the very *consciousness* of our cells, tissue and organs, which is what I have termed 'the physical soul'. For our cells themselves know of no other mode of experiencing *but* touch and taste, i.e.

tactile experiencing and what Samuel Avery calls 'chemical' experiencing on the other.

The radical conclusion that all these reflections inexorably lead to is that bodyhood as such *is* touch, i.e. *tactile experiencing* in general and *per se*.

The radical conclusion that all these reflections lead to is that bodyhood as such *is* touch, i.e. *tactile experiencing* in general and *per se*. It is not just that our bodies are an *instrument* or object of touch. Instead, the very 'body' that we think of as touching or being touched is, in itself, a felt shape or pattern *of* tactile experiencing.

It is not sight but *touch* then, that can be said to be the true essence of *all* sensory and bodily experiencing. Thus not only sensations of hardness and softness, roughness or softness, lightness or heaviness, weight and density, warmth and coolness but also of air and respiration, taste and digestion, lightness or heaviness, movement and stillness, tension and relaxation, sound and silence, even pleasure, pain and emotional states, that are felt in a principally *tactile* way; as also are such senses as 'pressure' of time, of spatial expansiveness or confinement, closeness or distance – not to mention our sense of how inwardly close or distant, 'in touch' or 'in contact' we feel with ourselves and others.

All that we see from the outside and call 'a body' is in essence nothing but a realm of actual and potential modes of tactile experiencing – proprioceptive and kinaesthetic, respiratory, auditory, olfactory (smell) or gustatory (taste and digestive sensations), emotional and relational. There are many people however, whose consciousness is so much dominated by sight that these dimensions of tactile experiencing may be almost totally subsumed by visual perception – by objects that are 'seen' in three-dimensional space - or, as they increasingly are, only as two-dimensional images on an electronic screen – including medical images created through CAT and MRI scans. One can link the general decline of tactile awareness and experiencing to the way in which screen technology has markedly accentuated a primary identification of the human body (not least the female body) with something 'seen', a mere visual image and to which the realm of actual or potential touch, whether in the form of handling objects or sexual touch, is either subordinated to or, in the case of both pornography and medical scans for example, made dependent upon. As a result, one may ask whether the very word 'body', with its immediate connotation of something seen in the form of a visual, mental or technological image, has itself become an obstacle to a more basic understanding of what 'a body' essentially *is*.

The same can be said of the word 'soul' – which is why I prefer the term 'feeling awareness'. In this context however, it is important to distinguish 'feeling' and 'touch'. If we touch something we of course 'feel' it. On the other hand we can be 'touched' in a feeling way and not just in the physical way *implied* by the term 'tactile' – just as feelings can also 'touch' us in a non-physical way. What we call 'soul', therefore, can be understood precisely as this *feeling* dimension of tactile experiencing.

To say that "the tactile realm of perception is the same thing as the body" is to say that not just what we call 'body' but *also* what we call 'soul' are, in essence, anything 'in the world' that we experience as 'touching' us in a manner that is *felt* in what may be more than just a 'tactile' way – whether this be a visual image or perception, a sensation of pleasure or pain, a look on a person's face or in their eyes, a sound, word or tone of voice, a painting, poem or piece of music – or a lived experience, event or encounter of any sort.

This is what makes it impossible to separate the 'lived body' and bodily self-experience from our lived or experienced world. For what most essentially constitutes our 'life world' *is* all that has the potential to touch us in a *feeling* way. Indeed any 'world' consists of nothing but particular potentials of felt, tactile experiencing – none of which arise from some 'thing' called 'the body' *or* 'the soul', but rather from 'feeling awareness' – an awareness which knows no bodily boundaries and yet is the essence of both 'body' *and* 'soul' – both of which consist essentially of felt shapes, patterns, tones and textures *of* awareness.

What we call 'a feeling' (singular noun) or 'feelings' (plural noun) is one thing. 'Feeling' (verb) on the other hand, is another. 'Feelings' are something we experience ourselves as 'having'. *Feeling* on the other hand is something we *do*. Or rather not something that 'we' do but that awareness itself 'does' – for without a feeling awareness of a self or selves – of an 'I', 'you', or 'we' – there could be no self or selves to experience, just as without a *feeling* awareness of *all* there is to potentially experience, there would be nothing to experience – and so also no field or felt world of experiencing, tactile or otherwise. The terms 'feeling awareness' and 'body of feeling awareness' therefore remain an important reminder that it is *not* the visually perceived and seemingly 'physical' or 'material' forms (cellular and bodily, thingly and worldly) that feel or touch, but rather *awareness itself* in all its different shapes, patterns, tones and textures – and that *what* awareness feels and 'touches' are essentially nothing but *other* such shapes and patterns, tones and textures *of* awareness.

Furthermore, since it is only through an *awareness* of experiencing that we first come to experience any 'self', 'body' or 'world' whatsoever, it follows that this awareness itself cannot – *in principle* – be the *property* or *product of* any self, body or world we are aware *of* – let alone enclosed within the apparent boundaries of what we *see* as 'a body' or 'brain'. This argument 'in principle', i.e. the recognition that awareness is fundamentally irreducible to any experienced phenomena – being itself the precondition or 'field condition' for experiencing in all its infinite modes and potentials – is what I call 'The Awareness Principle'.

Acknowledgements to Samuel Avery for his insights into the relation between visual and tactile dimensions of sensory experiencing and their relation to the myth of 'matter'.

References:
Avery, Samuel *The Dimensional Structure of Consciousness*
Avery, Samuel *Transcendence of the Western Mind* Wilberg, Peter *The Awareness Principle*

Appendices

1. Questions & Answers on Life Medicine – an Interview with Peter Wilberg

Ben Watt: Visits to the doctor often leave patients feeling marginalized and ignored. What has gone wrong?

Peter Wilberg: Doctors are 'trained' (indoctrinated in years-long boot camps might be a more appropriate way of putting it!) to reduce the human body to a *biological machine*. This training predisposes them *not* to see the patient's body as an embodied *self*, i.e. as the outer face of a *person* – and one whose 'inside' consists just as much of thoughts and feelings as of tissue and organs. The result is a total separation of biology from biography, the life of the human body from the life and life world of the individual human being. The body and its symptoms are not seen as a symbolic embodiment and expression of a dis-ease experienced in the patient's life (for example an experience of 'heartbreak' or total 'loss of heart' expressed as heart symptoms – or of childhood sexual abuse expressed as vaginal or anal symptoms). Instead of seeing the human body as an embodiment of the individual human being, it is treated as a mere 'thing' that the patient 'brings with them' to the doctor – like bringing a car to a garage. Unfortunately, many patients are already alienated or cut off from their own bodies, and may treat their own body as a mere thing or 'It' in the same way that many doctors do, thus colluding in a mutual 'We-It' relation to their illness.

Alternatively, however, patients will literally 'get ill to see a doctor' – turning a *life problem* into a *bodily symptom* just in order to get it at least medically recognised by another human being – and, through the specific and social role of the doctor, by society at large. But if the doctor fails to even try to see behind the patient's presenting symptoms – to see the life problems or distress they express and embody—the patient will indeed feel marginalised and ignored as a human being – as they will if they sense no authentic human warmth or empathy from their doctor. Michael Balint wrote of a 'collusion of anonymity' whereby patients are passed from one doctor or specialist to another without anyone *taking any interest in or responsibility for* the patient as a *person* – and one with a real life rather than just a name or hospital code number. Indeed, one consultant actually admitted to me that among his fellow professionals in the hospitals he worked in, patients *were not even referred to by their personal names*. Instead they were identified with their illness and referred to in a wholly impersonal way as 'The Emphysema' or 'The Liver Failure'.

This *depersonalisation* of the patient and their body is compounded by doctors' trained belief in maintaining 'clinical distance', i.e. to not show any human empathy whatsoever for the patient's lived experience of illness (for example of acute or chronic pain and the way this affects their lives. In the past, miners who developed chronic respiratory or back problems from having to work long shifts in almost airless tunnels not big enough to stand up straight in used to be told by their doctors: 'It's your work that's causing it – so get used to it'. Yet even today, doctors are still taught than any expression of subjective emotional *empathy* with patients is a threat to their clinical 'objectivity', rather than being central to the patient not feeling 'marginalised and ignored' – but instead fully taken in *as a unique person* with a unique life (and not just as 'somebody').

As regards human empathy or the lack of it, I myself recall an experience of mentioning an agonising seven-hour long attack of Trigeminal Neuralgia (known as the 'suicide disease' because it is one of the most painful illnesses known) to a clinical practitioner. But because for him it was a mere side-issue unrelated to my principal presenting symptom, there was literally *zero* empathic response – as if I'd just made some
280

totally inconsequential remark about the weather or traffic. In fact, so entrenched are they in their posture of 'clinical distance' that I have yet to hear one doctor whose *first words* in response to mine consisted of such basic, everyday empathic phrases such 'Sorry to hear that' or 'That sounds very distressing'.

Yet were doctors to truly take time to listen – *and also ask the right sort of questions,* for example, *'Is or has there been anything else bothering you in your life?',* a clear relation between what is really bothering the patient and life and their symptoms will often immediately pop out. Thus an elderly woman suffering from night-time heart pains—that the doctor initially only sees as possible signs of 'angina' requiring further clinical tests – may share (possibly for the first time) the continuing *heartache* she feels from recently losing her husband – and losing him to a *night-time heart* attack at that. Or else a patient with a chronically aching shoulder might be found to answer 'Yeah, since my cousin/brother/business partner pulled out of our business I feel I've had to *shoulder* everything – and I mean everything – on my own'. Many more examples and case studies of symptoms as a type of 'somatic metaphor' for feelings and life problems are given on my site.

Ben Watt: Could you distinguish your approach to human suffering and illness from that currently prevalent in healthcare?

Peter Wilberg: A whole range of sharp differences between conventional biological medicine on the one hand, and what I call 'Existential Medicine' or 'Life Medicine' on the other are summarised in a two-column table on my website. One of the most basic answers to your question however, as suggested by the very title of my book, lies in its recognition that illness and suffering have an innately healing or 'curative' value and purpose in themselves. In other words, instead of seeing illness as something to be cured, the Life Doctoring recognises illness itself as the cure – our body's way of calling upon us and helping to change ourselves, our lives and our world. Thus simply asking ourselves and recognising what an illness is *stopping* us from doing (for example, overworking) can offer a key to its healing purpose, as can the recognition of what it may be forcing us to do (to take more for ourselves for example). But no illness will have the same *meaning* for every individual, and it is this individually curative life *meaning* – and not a more or less individual 'cause' or 'cure' of the biological or genetic sort – that Life Doctoring serves to help the patient to discover on many levels – and in its many, often complex individual aspects.

A central metaphor I employ in my writings to get over this new approach is the idea of illness as *a form of pregnancy* – in other words, a process of *gestating, giving birth to and learning to embody new and different aspects of ourselves* – and with them a new and different way of 'being in the world' and of of living our lives. That process – like pregnancy itself – can of course require much time – whether weeks, months, or, in certain cases of chronic illness, many years or even a whole lifetime. With this metaphor of 'illness as pregnancy' in mind much medical treatment is really aimed at using drugs or surgery to terminate the patient's pregnancy. Which is why treatments for serious illness, even when successful, are often followed by the patient developing another illness – or the same illness again. One can also compare see illnesses as 'body dreams' – or rather as 'body nightmares'. Were it possible that medicine had the technology to scan a patient's dreams, what would happen if a nightmarish monster were discovered in them? No doubt this monster would be regard as the principal 'cause' of the patient's nightmares. Perhaps, then, the same dream-scanning technology could be used to 'censor' the patient's dreams and prevent any possibility of the monster appearing again – an equivalent to surgically removing a tumour. Yet would doing so in any way explain or deal with the reasons for the patient's having this monstrous nightmare (or tumour) in the first place? Comparing illnesses to body dreams and nightmares allows us to see just how *backward* modern biological medicine really is – comparable in its view of illnesses to the way a lot of people, in particular scientists, thought of dreams in the era before Freud, i.e. seeing them as completely *meaningless* experiences rather than as having deep personal life meanings.

Ben Watt: What is the wheat and the chaff of biological medicine

Peter Wilberg: Another good question – though behind and in answer to it is the question of what *doctors themselves* regard as 'wheat' and what as 'chaff'. If the patient's life as a whole – including their life problems, stresses or dilemmas, current or recent life circumstances and events, life history and experiences and their most important life relationships are all regarded as 'chaff', then even to speak of 'biological' medicine is a contradiction in terms – the root Greek meaning of the modern term 'biology' being 'the speech' (*logos*) of 'life' (*bios*)'. It is the way in which difficult and often painful – but at the same time deep and potentially transformative – aspects of our *life* themselves *speak* through our bodies and through illness – as they also speak through our dreams—that constitutes what should be the 'wheat' of 'biological medicine '. Thus if a patient felt or feels 'stifled' or 'unable to breathe' in their *life* – for example, in their home or place of work, their family or particular relationships, or in particular places or life circumstances, is it enough to simply diagnose some disease entity called 'asthma' and give them inhalers for the rest of their life? If another patient feels subconsciously *inflamed* with anger at some person or situation in his or her life, what help is it to simply diagnose and treat the resulting inflammation of their skin or another biological organ? If someone finds a situation or person in their lives 'a pain in the ass', is it enough to perform a rectal examination and look for sensitive haemorrhoids? If the same children 'known' to be reactive to a particular allergen can be *unknowingly* exposed to it in a clinical environments – *and yet show no allergic reaction to it of the sort they do at home or in school* – then what is it their bodies are really reacting to through their 'allergy'? The list of questions such as these is endless, and the possible answers all highly individual and therefore infinitely variable. And yet precisely because they cannot be compiled into a neat set of statistics or pinned down to some particular gene it is biological medicine itself that discards them as 'chaff'.

Ben Watt: Many people believe that biological medicine has proven itself with such achievements as surgery under anesthesia, antibiotics, vaccines, and genetic analysis. Do you disagree, and if so, why?

Peter Wilberg: These 'achievements' *may* be regarded as another element of the 'wheat' in biological medicine, its 'good stuff'—although, taking each of the achievements in turn, one can find many good reasons for disagreement.

1. *Surgery under anaesthesia.* I have already referred to the principal natural sources, not just of most modern pain relievers but also anaesthetics. As for surgery as such, putting aside emergency surgery for war or accident injuries, stroke or heart attack victims etc., there remains the larger question of meaning—of how and why people come to *require surgery* – for whatever reason, in the first place. Or rather the question is, in what ways might a *life- and meaning-based approach to medicine* have prevented or forestalled the need for surgery ever arising? Conversely, why is it that, even according to the medical research itself, so much wholly unnecessary and/or damaging and counter-productive surgery is performed? A principal reason is that patients' needs are assessed according to *statistical risk factors* and not as those of individuals. That is why so many women have had a breast removed only to find there was no cancer there, or that so many men have been

rendered impotent and/or incontinent, not just by surgical treatment but simply through *surgical testing* for prostate cancer – conducted solely on the basis of dubious *statistical* risks of prostate cancer based on how much of a particular antigen they have in their blood.

2. *Antibiotics.* Five points. Firstly, antibiotics treatments developed grew out of the accidental discovery of the bacterial effects of a naturally occurring mould or fungus – not through some pharmaceutical company designing a molecule unknown in nature or to the human body. Secondly, the widespread use of antibiotics did not develop until after major epidemic infections declined as a result of improved hygiene and sanitation. Thirdly, as we know, the overuse of antibiotics threatens to render the bacilli they were designed to treat ever more resistant. Fourthly, though I have been as grateful for the availability of antibiotics as many others, their successful use has not in any way explained why the medical conditions requiring their use arose in the first place – nor prevented their repeated use for the same or other conditions. Only a *meaning-based* approach to the medical conditions most often treated with antibiotics can explain this. For fifthly, since we all constantly carry the bacteria which supposedly 'cause' sore throats – and a host of other illnesses, including lethal ones – we should at least *all have sore throats all the time* and *be in constant need of antibiotics* to treat them. So what other factors in our lives and psyches prevent this happening?

3. *Vaccines.* Many very big questions about these too – too many to go into here. But as with antibiotics some of the questions never fully addressed are what makes certain people susceptible to a particular bacillus *or* virus in the first place, and how come many people come in contact with them without getting ill at all – even during plagues and epidemics? Another question is whether their use might not make the body *less able* to distinguish a potentially threatening virus from a harmless one contained in a vaccine. Even many

doctors argue that better specific and general immunity is created by actually contracting certain childhood illnesses than by vaccinating against them. Finally, we have yet to explain why the incidence of polio, for example, was already falling before mass vaccination was introduced. Finally, there are many who would claim, with good reasons, that the multiple constituents of most vaccines are in themselves *highly toxic*.

4. *Genetic medicine*. It is one thing to recognise that, far from being a mere biological machine, the human body is a living biological *language* of the human being—and that illness too is a form of body language and bodily communication. It is *quite another thing* however, to reduce this language to genetic strings of molecules constituting our DNA. The huge danger new forms of genetic medicine threatens us with come from the belief that we can remove or disable genes associated with a particular disease *with no other effects resulting*. This is rather like thinking we can eliminate the use of 'bad' language by simply censoring or removing from our linguistic vocabulary certain sequences of sounds and letters these 'bad' words contain. The claims made by genetic medicine are in some ways philosophically quite infantile—as if some genius has discovered that – WOW! – the words *yuck, muck, fuck* and *sucks* – all contain the letter sequence *u-c-k*. So we'll just take a sequence like *u-c-k* out of your genetic vocabulary – and good *l-u-c-k* to you!

Ben Watt: What thoughts do you have on alternative medicine and the other practitioners who describe themselves as holistic?

Peter Wilberg: Many if not most forms of alternative medicine follow exactly the same basic model as orthodox medicine, seeing illness and health as opposites, and seeking *causes and cures* for a patient's illness, rather than seeking to understand its *meaning* and *healing value* in the larger context of their lives. It makes no difference whether you see a patient's illness as 'caused' by an energy block, evil spirit, virus, mutated cell or gene – the basic model is the same.

The only difference is one of *language*. Thus a practitioner of New Age 'energy medicine' for example, might 'diagnose' an illness as a result of an 'energy block' in one or more of the patient's 'chakras'. Similarly, practitioners of traditional forms of Chinese and Indian Ayurvedic medicine differ only in employing very different diagnostic and even anatomical *vocabularies* to those of modern Western biological medicine (see my essays and book chapters on 'Alternative Medicine' and 'Energy Medicine').

I myself actually avoid the word 'holistic' in describing my work, used as it so often is today in a way that implies that the human being is precisely *not* a unitary whole – inseparable from their life and life world as a whole – but rather a mere assemblage of *separable parts* labelled 'Body, Mind, and Spirit' (and in this sense no different *in essence* from any other assemblage such as a car).

Ben Watt: So, to recapitulate, what are doctors for?

Peter Wilberg: A very good question indeed! Indeed, in a recent essay of mine entitled *Automated Diagnosis and the Future of Biomedicine*, I pose the question of what essentially a doctor is *doing* while listening to a patient. I argue that if what the doctor is doing is essentially going through a sort of calculative 'algorithm' or 'decision tree' in order to end up with one or more possible diagnoses, then the doctor could just as well be replaced by *automated diagnostic software systems* – built on a far larger and more up-to-date databases of symptom clusters and diseases, and incorporating far more detailed and integrated patient medical records, than any human doctor could possibly 'store' in their own head. On the other hand, the availability and increased use of computer assisted diagnosis could also potentially also free the doctor from the role of serving as a mere *human medical computer* – a 'black box' between the patient's 'input' and some form of mentally computed 'output' in the form of prescriptions, further tests, or referrals to specialists. Instead they could give their full attention to exploring the symbolic life meaning of a patient's symptoms – and even the very symbolism to be found in the scientific terminologies used to account for them. For we must not forget that what is seen as medical 'science' is as much based on metaphor as on 'facts' or 'evidence' (for example, the *military* metaphor of 'counter-attacks' by immunological 'defenses' against colonising 'foreign bodies', in the form of microorganisms, cancerous cells, etc). And the whole notion of illnesses – not least cancer – as something against which a war must be fought pervades the mindset of most doctors and their patients, even though not a single form of expensively researched and 'aggressive' hi-tech treatment for cancer, though a source of huge profits for the health industry, has been shown to increase the life expectancy of cancer patients (though such treatments, whether through surgery, chemo- or radiotherapy do often devastate the patient's *quality of life*). Yet the single word 'cancer' has become a symbol of how not just doctors but most people now understands illness – as a type of *invasion or colonisation* by mutant cells or 'foreign' bodies of all sorts. Indeed, in this sense, the word 'cancer' has become the *medical equivalent* of derogatory terms for Jews and Blacks.

Coming back to the question however, our notion of what doctors *are for* has also come a long way from a time – only a few centuries ago – when the use of even simple measuring instruments such as thermometers was regarded as quackery, as was the very notion of 'diagnosing' some sort of hidden disease 'entity' causing the patients symptoms. At that time emphasis was still placed on providing both *symptomatic relief* to patients – whether in the form of human care and comfort, *wise and healing words*, or natural plant remedies such like willow bark or the seeds of the poppy plant – which *still* represent the principal natural raw material for profitable pharmaceutically-patented pain-relieving drugs such as 'aspirin' (a constituent of willow bark), codeine and morphine, as well anaesthetics such as novocaine.

'I don't care what you know unless I know that you care.' This saying offers another answer to the question of why many patients are unhappy with the sort of treatment they get from doctors—or rather the way medical treatment has replaced authentically human health *care*. Michael Balint wrote of the 'drug' that we call 'doctor'. It is the degree and depth of *life experience and empathic life understanding* that the patient feels coming from a particular doctor – as expressed in his or her way of listening, words, body language, general demeanour and manner of communication – that has the most powerful and immediate effect on the patient's sense of well-being – or the very opposite. In other words it is to the *doctor-patient relationship* and the nature of *doctor-patient communication* that we should look in addressing the big question: *What are doctors are for?* Currently, however, it is as if the patient as a human being does not even figure in medical discourse at all. Thus, one can read literally thousands of 'scientific' and supposedly 'evidence-based' medical research papers *in none of which can be found so much as single reference* to the patient's lived experience of illness, their experience of the particular form of surgery or treatment described – or often even to the *symptoms* that it was intended to treat! In general, 'successful' treatment is more and more equated to observed changes in a *visual representation* of the patient's body, whether through numbers on a chart or images from a X-ray or scanning device – and that irrespective of whether the patient *actually experiences any improvement in their symptoms*. The result can be tragi-comic. For as a friend of mine shared with me, he himself was told – *without even a hint of irony* – that the surgical procedure conducted on his father had been

completely 'successful' – aside from the minor detail that his father had died during the operation. The side-effects of medical drugs and surgery as actually experienced by patients are almost never reported in medical journals and papers, but are just ignored as a form of 'collateral damage' that the patient has to put up with. Reading *patient experience forums* on the Internet however (something it seems doctors never do) tells us quite a different story – often offering a host of horror stories recounting the distressing, often chronic or even permanently *life-damaging* effects of different types of medical drug or surgery.

Ben Watt: In the light of your thinking, how do you help the ill who come to your home?

Peter Wilberg: Like many counsellors today, I do not only see clients at home but also engage with them through correspondence and Skype. Nor do I see Life Doctoring, i.e. counselling for serious illness – as a replacement for consultations with ordinary doctor, but as a necessary complement to conventional doctoring – that is until medical training itself begins to turn out doctors already steeped in the basic philosophy of 'Life Medicine'. As for the patient, first contact is usually made by phone or e-mail enquiry. In response I invariably request that a potential patient writes to me again, but this time attaching (a) as detailed a medical history as possible, including of course an account of their current medical condition and its history – along with any drugs they are or have been on on or any treatments that they have received or that have been suggested to them (b) as detailed an account also of their *life history* as they are prepared to offer – including whatever life circumstance, events and experiences, as well as family and other relationships, they consider as having been most important.

Finally, I might also suggest that they *begin* to answer in writing also some of the questions listed in my book and on my site under the title What Most Doctors Don't Ask. These questions are then followed up in face to face sessions and/or through phone or Skype calls and further correspondence – for they are central in beginning to gain valuable insight into 'the hidden story' behind a patient's illness, i.e. the ways in which difficulties in their lives may be symbolised by their symptoms (see also Brian Broom: *Somatic Illness and the Patient's Other Story*). For this purpose however, it is of the utmost importance that the Life Doctor be as *medically informed as possible* of the specific nature of the patient's condition – whether through very competent and thorough research skills, by virtue of already being a doctor, or through consultation with medical professionals and specialists. Only in this way can they help a patient in *all the many ways* that I see as defining the principal aims of Life Doctoring – both as new and specialist form of counselling (for serious illness) and as a new approach to 'doctoring' itself. For it must not be forgotten that though not necessarily a conventionally trained or 'qualified' doctor, the Life Doctor not only has additional and very important skills, to ordinary doctors, but also a different *type* of knowledge of illness – and indeed of the nature of the human body as such – knowledge of a sort most conventional doctors *do not* get from their training.

With this in mind, the overall helping aims and methods of my work as Life Doctor can be briefly summarised as follows:

- Giving patients the opportunity to share their experience of illness *in all its life dimensions* – not least its subjective, social, emotional and relational dimensions. This includes the opportunity to express their experience of medical practitioners and services and/or voice their concerns around specific medical diagnoses, prognoses and treatments.

- Giving patients greater quantity and quality of *listening* time – not just a rushed seven, ten or even twenty minute consultation but anything from 1 to 4 *hours* of deep, patient and empathic listening. True healing can only begin with the patient being *fully heard* and given the time also to be fully 'heard out' beyond the confines of what are generally absurdly limited time boundaries.

- Well-researched and individually tailored advice in making *informed choices* about proposed medical tests and treatments, based on knowledge of their potential dangers and side-effects – and alternatives to them. It is important that the Life Doctor be able to protect patients from being persuaded into accepting potentially dangerous, counter-productive or even life-threatening forms of orthodox biomedical treatment, as well as to advise and support them in preparing for consultations with their doctors, consultants, surgeons or other health professionals.

- Teaching patients ways to more deeply reflect on and *meditate* their symptoms – including pain – rather than just *medicating* those symptoms. In this way – and through the Life Doctor's own *highly trained* therapeutic and body awareness – helping patients to uncover the *life story* behind their illness – its biographical as well as 'medical' history, its symbolic meaning in the context of their lives and its potentially *healing value* in transforming their lives.

- This means helping patients to *retrace and reverse the process* by which they turned particular life relationships, life experiences and life problems *into illnesses* – and instead begin to approach those life experiences, life problems and life relationships anew, with a fresh awareness and from a fresh perspective, whilst at the same time always offering the patient on-going emotional support in just coping with their illness and suffering on an everyday basis.

2. Biomedical Psychiatry – A Health Warning

Your symptoms – or those of your clients or patients if you are a counsellor or doctor – may themselves be effects of the very drugs that are being or have been prescribed to 'treat' them.

Recent decades have seen an enormous rise in the number of people treated with psychopharmaceutical medications – all of which have a direct effect on brain functioning. Such medications include:

Antidepressants (in particular so-called SSRI's which raise serotonin levels in the brain)

Anxiolytics (for treating anxiety, sleep problems and panic attacks – in particular the large range of so-called benzodiazepines such as Valium)

Neuroleptics (for treating so-called psychotic symptoms)

Stimulants (used on an increasing scale to treat children and adults with so-called behaviour disorders such as Attention Deficit Disorder)

Anticonvulsants (usually prescribed for epilepsy, fibromyalgia and neuralgias but some of which, for example pregabalin, are also prescribed for anxiety disorders)

What is not so well known is that many of the psychological and somatic symptoms treated by counsellors and psychotherapists, physicians and psychiatrists are a direct result of taking or having taken medications of these sorts. Symptoms such as depression, anxiety, sleep disturbances, panic attacks, phobias, compulsions, mania, poor concentration, loss of affect, suicidal thoughts and psychotic episodes are all recognised by pharmaceutical companies themselves as potential effects of the very medications designed to treat them. Indeed it has been estimated that up to 50% of all patients attending mental health services may be presenting with anxiety disorders resulting from the use of anxiety-treating drugs or 'anxiolytics' – specifically the benzodiazepines. This is due to the development of dependency and acute or chronic withdrawal symptoms – such as increased anxiety or panic attacks – even whilst taking prescribed doses, whose efficacy declines as neuro-physiological habituation to the drugs or 'tolerance' sets in.

According to the psychiatrist Peter Breggin, health practitioners now confront a hidden epidemic of *iatrogenic* (medically caused) psychical and somatic illness resulting from short or long-term chemical disruption of brain functioning. The adverse effects of psychopharmaceutical medications, both acute and chronic, include:

- intended effects (for example the mind-numbing depression of brain functioning and the dulling of thought and emotion induced by *neuroleptics*).

- paradoxical effects (accentuation of the very symptoms which the drugs were prescribed to treat, such as panic attacks induced by *anxiolytics*).

- physiological side effects (ranging from respiratory, cardiac, gastrointestinal problems to long-term brain and liver damage, peripheral nerve damage, sexual dysfunction, weight gain, chronic fatigue or dyskinesia (uncontrolled Parkinsonian-type movements).

- psychological side effects (symptoms of mania, depression, panic attacks, psychotic episodes, suicidal ideation etc. of a sort not previously experienced by the individual at any time before taking the medications).

- withdrawal effects (acute or chronic psychological and physiological effects experienced when coming off prescribed medications).

- tolerance effects (needing ever-increasing dosages of the same drug to simply avoid what can be acute and frequent inter-dose withdrawal effects).

- short and long-term 'dependency' (in plain language addiction – resulting in tolerance and need for ever-higher doses to avoid withdrawal symptoms.)

There is a tendency to interpret even the most dangerous physiological side-effects – if reported – merely as symptoms of a patient's psychological disorder. Cardiac symptoms, for example, may be interpreted as 'anxiety' symptoms, rather than the other way round. As a result, patients with genuine cardiac problems may remain medically untested and untreated until they suffer a serious heart attack.

Many social workers, nurses and even GPs, counsellors, psychotherapists and alternative health practitioners however, still believe that the use and efficacy of psychopharmaceutical drugs is scientifically proven. The medical myth has it that mental disorders such as 'depression' are caused by biochemical imbalances in the brain. Not only has there never been any scientific evidence of this whatsoever, it is actually not technically possible to measure the levels of neurotransmitters in the synapses between brain cells. The hypothesis of an original 'chemical imbalance' was arrived at by arguing backwards from the supposedly therapeutic effects of drugs designed to chemically influence the release or reuptake of particular neurotransmitters – thereby altering their respective levels in the brain, even though the latter cannot be directly measured. Thus whilst there is no evidence that such drugs correct imbalances in the brain, they can be chemically guaranteed to cause them – artificially elevating or depressing neurotransmitter levels in a way that may affect not only mood, but all the body's most basic regulatory systems.

The principal 'evidence' for the therapeutic efficacy of psychopharmaceutical medications comes from short-term clinically controlled studies comparing the effects of an active drug with that of an inactive or 'inert' placebo. In most cases, the difference between the drug and placebo thought necessary to scientifically 'prove' the efficacy of the former is minimal. But comparing the effects of any active drug with an inert placebo is, as Peter Breggin says, misleading in itself. This is because the active drug may have its own type of placebo effect – giving the patient a felt sense of a drug's power by virtue of its felt effects, however subtle.

As John Grohol points out:

"...the double-blind placebo controlled study is not blind. Side effects are so obvious that more than 80% of the patients know whether they are on active medication or placebo, patients are equally accurate about other patients on the ward, and nurses and other personnel are privy as well. In some studies the only people who claim to be blind are the prescribing physicians, and in other studies the prescribing physicians admit being as aware of the patients' condition as everyone else." Even with active placebos *"the empirical data show that medication effect sizes are hard to distinguish from the placebo. Also not mentioned is that most antidepressant medications habituate, and the patients' symptoms return. Most patients believe they would feel even worse if they were not taking their medication."*

Grohol goes on to question the use of clinician-rated rather than patient-rated measures of 'improvement' in such trials, noting that:

"If patients cannot tell that they are better off in a controlled study, one must question the conventional wisdom about the efficacy of antidepressant drugs."

One of the main arguments in favour of the use of anti-depressants is suicide and violence prevention. How is it then, that several studies have shown an actual increase in suicide rates in those taking anti-depressants? How is that otherwise sober and responsible individuals with no history of violence or severe personality disorder can, within a few day or weeks fall victim to violent or suicidal impulses, even to the point of committing murder or suicide? One reason is the stimulant effect of the new Prozac-type antidepressants or Selective Serotonin Reuptake Inhibitors (SSRIs). The artificially elevated serotonin levels they are designed to induce can result not only in mild euphoria but manic states or psychotic syndromes similar to those produced by illegal amphetamines. Alternatively, they may, in the first few days of usage, result in an unnatural depression of serotonin levels as the brain tries to compensate for an artificially induced chemical imbalance. In both cases the drug has brought about a form of organic brain dysfunction of the very sort assumed, without evidence, to be responsible for the patient's symptoms. Another argument for the use of anti-depressants is their 'efficacy' for many people. No thought is given however, as to the reasons why such drugs are felt or deemed to be 'effective'. Breggin explains that:

"A patient typically is rendered unable to stay depressed during an episode of organic brain dysfunction, because depression requires a relatively intact brain and mind. Rendered either apathetic or artificially euphoric by brain dysfunction, the patient is evaluated as 'improved'."

"What psychiatrists call 'depression' – lethargy, apathy, nervousness, hopelessness, helplessness and unhappiness – is a serious problem often unrecognised as drug-related. Because of their depressant and debilitating effect, psychiatric drugs can make people feel so bad they want to kill themselves."

SSRI's such as *paroxetine* (Seroxat/Paxil) and Prozac may be authorised for use by patients over many years on the basis of clinical trials lasting from only 6 to 10 weeks. GlaxoSmithKline, whose sales of Seroxat/Paxil were valued at over one and a half billion pounds in 2000, continue aggressive marketing of the drug to doctors, with 100 million prescriptions given annually. This despite the fact that their own staff reported trial patients showing significant withdrawal symptoms of agitation and insomnia after only a short period on the drug – which now leads the World Health Organisation's list of pharmaceuticals reported by doctors to cause acute withdrawal problems. GSK leaflet accompanying prescriptions still tell the patient that "you cannot become addicted to Seroxat." No distinction is made between dependency of the sort comparable to an addict's cravings for tobacco or heroin, and addiction based purely on the need to avoid acute physical or psychological withdrawal symptoms.

The information leaflet for Seroxat also includes the following words:

"Occasionally, the symptoms of depression may include thoughts of harming yourself or committing suicide. Until the full antidepressant effect of your medication becomes apparent it is possible that these symptoms may increase in the first few weeks of treatment."

The tone is soothing. But in June 2001, GSK were forced to pay out $6.4 million in damages to the family of a man who killed his wife, daughter, granddaughter and then himself after only two days on Seroxat.

In contrast to the SSRIs, most *neuroleptic* drugs or 'anti-psychotics', together with the minor and major tranquillizers, work by dulling and depressing brain activity through a wide range of different neurotransmitters including dopamine and GABA. The artificially-induced elevation or depression of mood brought on by the elevation or depression of different neurotransmitters in the brain, may have dramatic effects when the drug is *withdrawn* – either producing a dramatic 'rebound' elevation of neurotransmitter levels or leaving the brain incapable of generating normal neurotransmitter levels by itself. Breggin cites a typical example of withdrawal syndrome:

"Recently one of my patients, a young man in his twenties, was trying to taper off small doses of Elavil prescribed by another physician...within a day or two of complete withdrawal he began to feel ill. It seemed exactly like the flu. He felt lethargic and his muscles ached. He lacked appetite, felt sick to his stomach, and vomited in the morning.

Despite his tiredness he had trouble falling asleep and staying asleep. He felt increasing anxiety as well. A complete physical examination by an internist revealed no evidence of an infection, and I was forced to conclude that he had a typical flu-like withdrawal syndrome. He gradually recovered over a few weeks, vomiting for the last time about a month after ending the medication."

Not all are so 'lucky' as this patient. Countless harrowing stories by those who became unknowingly dependent on highly-addictive *benzodiazepine* tranquillizers and sleeping pills, or so-called 'non-addictive' anti-depressants, bear testament to the years or even decades of hell suffered in the attempt to withdraw from these drugs, and/or of the permanent post-withdrawal symptoms they still suffer.

With one out of four people in the UK thought to be suffering from a diagnosable mental disorder, the number of prescriptions of anti-depressants and anxiolytics is vast.

As long ago as 1984, it was reported by Professor Malcolm Lader that 11.2 percent of all adults took a *benzodiazepine* for anxiety or sleeping problems in any one year.

According to Lader:

'Even at a conservative estimate, 20% of these will develop symptoms when they attempt to withdraw. That means a quarter of a million people in the UK. It is now estimated that one and a half million people in the UK alone are chronically addicted to benzodiazepine anxiolytics such as diazepam (Valium) and lorazepam (Ativan). All the drugs in this class can induce dependency in a matter of days through suppressing the brain 's natural production of anxiety- and stress-reducing neurotransmitters. Yet they account for 50% of global sales of psychopharmaceutical medications.'

Benzodiazepine use can also cause numerous *physical* health problems such as dental pains, abdominal disorders, acute neuralgias, muscle aches and a whole host of other symptoms – all of which may be misdiagnosed and mistreated by dentists, physicians and consultants unaware of this.

The whole situation was summed up by Vernon Coleman (*Life Without Tranquillizers*)

"The biggest drug-addiction problem in the world doesn't involve heroin, cocaine or marijuana. In fact, it doesn't involve an illegal drug at all. The world's biggest drug-addiction problem is posed by a group of drugs, the benzodiazepines, which are widely prescribed by doctors and taken by countless millions of perfectly ordinary people around the world... Drug-addiction experts claim that getting people off the benzodiazepines is more difficult than getting addicts off heroin... For several years now pressure-groups have been fighting to help addicted individuals break free from their pharmacological chains. But the fight has been a forlorn one. As fast as one individual breaks free from one of the benzodiazepines another patient somewhere else becomes addicted. I believe that the main reason for this is that doctors are addicted to prescribing benzodiazepines just as much as patients are hooked on taking them."

The sheer scale of the problem with psychopharmaceutical medications becomes clear if we consider that probably 75% or more of so-called 'adverse reactions', including withdrawal symptoms and withdrawal syndromes, may be unreported. Worse still, they may be unrecognised as such by patients themselves, interpreted as signs of endogenous psychological disorders by physicians or psychotherapists, and/or treated by prescriptions of further psychiatric drugs. In an attempt to deal with recognised side-effects of these drugs, many psychiatrists and psychiatric health clinics around the world now regularly prescribe whole 'cocktails' of anti-depressant, neuroleptic and anxiolytic medications in the hope that they will chemically counter-balance each other's inherently toxic and unbalancing effects on brain functioning. At the same time pharmaceutical companies such as GSK are inventing ever new 'disorders' which can be 'treated' by drugs such as paroxetine. As well as 'panic disorder', 'obsessive compulsive disorder' the list now includes 'post-traumatic stress disorder' and 'social anxiety disorder' and 'attention deficit disorder'. Yet like standard DSM psychiatric designations such as 'bipolar disorder', 'personality disorder', these new 'disorder' terms seem to possess the authority of medical diagnoses – implying the existence of specific disease entities with an organic basis. In fact they are merely convenient labels for clusters of troublesome symptoms or behaviours that society has a problem understanding and responding to.

Biological psychiatry is founded on a flat denial that there is any meaning in 'mental illness', ignoring the simple fact that in a sick society or economy there may be good reasons for a person to feel anxious, depressed, disturbed, divided or driven to compulsive behaviours in order to cope. Illnesses in general are regarded as having biological 'causes' rather than meanings related to the individual's life.

Health itself is essentially defined only as the ability to 'function' normally as an employee – to cheerfully play one's part in sustaining a market economy in which all human relations are geared solely to commodity production and profit making. As a result, both medicine and psychiatry have both become tools of the 'therapeutic state' – their principal role being to manage or suppress all bodily or behavioural symptoms of the distress and dis-ease engendered by a sick society, not least with the help of drugs – thereby also turning them into a lucrative source of profit for the corporate health industry.

'Authoritarian psychiatry' is now being legitimised by governments all over the world through legislation, which denies mental patients the right to refuse medication and permits their enforced detention and drug 'treatment '. Given the enormous attention given by politicians and the media to the problems caused by illegal drugs and drug addiction, the failure by governments and health services to recognise the scale of addiction to legally prescribed drugs and the dangers of their adverse effects is hypocritical to say the least – amounting to a form of wilful ignorance. It is all the more important then, that social workers, mental health nurses, counsellors, psychotherapists and alternative health practitioners do not fall into the trap that so many orthodox physicians and psychiatrists have fallen into – that of accepting the medical and marketing myths perpetuated by pharmaceutical companies regarding the 'benefits' of psychiatric medications. Above all, it is important that they:

- obtain precise details of any client's present or past use, not only of illegal drugs but of legally prescribed medications, including the names of these medications and the length of time over which they were or have been taken.

- educate themselves in the adverse effects, addictive potentials and withdrawal symptoms of specific anxiolytic, anti-depressant and neuroleptic medications.

Thankfully, use of the internet now allows any patient or professional to quickly obtain information regarding specific drugs and drug types, as well as being host to many websites set up to support patients suffering from adverse reactions or dependency on such drugs, to inform health professionals of their dangers, to advise both patients and practitioners on safe methods of withdrawal, or simply to provide a forum in which users can share with each other the often horrifying experiences they have had of particular medications and their debilitating or life-destroying effects.

Recommended sites

benzohelp.blogspot.com
www.benzo.org.uk - info on benzodiazepines
www.quitpaxil.org - info on paroxetine (Paxil/Seroxat)
www.breggin.com - excellent articles by Peter Breggin
www.antipsychiatry.org - the case against biopsychiatry
www.april.org.uk - on adverse drug reactions
www.citawithdrawal.org.uk - Council for Information on Tranquillisers, Antidepressants and Painkillers

Recommended Reading

- Peter R. Breggin *Toxic Psychiatry*
- Breggin / Cohen *Your Drug May be Your Problem*
- Joan E. Gadsby *Addiction by Prescription*
- Heather Jones *Prisoner on Prescription*
- David Smail *The Nature of Unhappiness*
- Dr Ann Tracy *Prozac - Panacea or Pandora*

3. Death by Doctoring

"In the United States – where 40,000 people are shot to death each year – the chance of getting "killed" by a doctor is three times greater than being killed by a gun." Ben Ong

"An article written by Dr Barbara Starfield, MD, MPH, of the John Hopkins School of Hygiene and Public Health, shows that medical errors may be the third leading cause of death in the United States. The report apparently shows there are 2,000 deaths/year from unnecessary surgery ; 7000 deaths/year from medication errors in hospitals; 20,000 deaths/year from other errors in hospitals; 80,000 deaths/year from infections in hospitals; 106,000 deaths/year from non-error, adverse effects of medications – these total up to 225,000 deaths per year in the US from iatrogenic causes which ranks these deaths as the third killer. Iatrogenic is a term used when a patient dies as a direct result of treatments by a physician, whether it is from misdiagnosis of the ailment or from adverse drug reactions used to treat the illness (drug reactions are the most common cause). Based on the findings of one major study, medical errors kill some 44,000 people in U.S. hospitals each year. Another study puts the number much higher, at 98,000. Even using the lower estimate, more people die from medical mistakes each year than from highway accidents, breast cancer, or AIDS. And deaths from medication errors that take place both in and out of hospitals are said to be more than 7,000 annually." www.cancure.org/medical_errors.htm

Indeed the statistics point to medicine actually being the first and leading cause of death. For in the 2001 annual death rate from heart disease in the U.S. was 699,697; and the cancer death rate was 553,251.

Compare this with the following table for 'iatrogenic' or medically induced deaths:

Adverse Drug Reactions	106,000
Medical error	98,000
Bedsores	115,000
Infection	88,000
Malnutrition	108,800
Outpatients	199,000
Unnecessary Procedures	37,136
Total	**783,936**

Projected over a ten-year period this gives us a figure of almost 7.84 million – more than all the deaths from all the wars fought by America. Note also the projected ten-year statistics for 'unnecessary events' i.e. unnecessary medical intervention, along with the corresponding figures for adverse results stemming from these unnecessary treatment 'procedures'.

Unnecessary Events

Hospitalization	89 million	17 million
Procedures	75 million	15 million
TOTAL	164 million	

As Ben Ong notes, this table indicates that *56% of the population of the United States, have been treated unnecessarily by the medical industry* – in other words, nearly 50,000 people per day.

ben.ong@cure-prostate.com

"The National Academies website published an article titled "Preventing Death and Injury From Medical Errors Requires Dramatic, System-Wide Changes." which you can read online at 'www4.nationalacademies.org/news.nsf/isbn/0309068371?O penDocument' or the book "To Err Is Human: Building a Safer Health System" at www.nap.edu/books/0309068371/html/ – These show medical errors as a leading cause of death. Based on the findings of one major study, medical errors kill some 44,000 people in U.S. hospitals each year. Another study puts the number much higher, at 98,000. Even using the lower estimate, more people die from medical mistakes each year than from highway accidents, breast cancer, or AIDS. And deaths from medication errors that take place both in and out of hospitals are said to be more than 7,000 annually."

Reference:
www.cancure.org/medical_errors.htm

4. Prescription Drugs – Leading Killer in USA

"... a statistical study of hospital deaths in the U.S. conducted at the University of Toronto revealed that pharmaceutical drugs kill more people every year than are killed in traffic accidents. The study is said to show that more than two million American hospitalized patients suffered a serious adverse drug reaction (ADR) within the 12-month period of the study and, of these, over 100,000 died as a result. The researchers found that over 75 per cent of these ADRs were dose-dependent, which suggests they were due to the inherent toxicity of the drugs rather than to allergic reactions.

The data did not include fatal reactions caused by accidental overdoses or errors in administration of the drugs. If these had been included, it is estimated that another 100,000 deaths would be added to the total every year. The researchers concluded that ADRs are now the fourth leading cause of death in the United States after heart disease, cancer, and stroke."

www.cancure.org/medical_errors.htm

"Getting the wrong drug or the wrong dosage kills hundreds or thousands of people each year, with many times that number getting injured ... Even higher than the number of people who die from medication errors is the number of people who die from medication, period. Even when a prescription drug is dispensed properly, there's no guarantee it won't end up killing you. A remarkable study in the Journal of the American Medical Association revealed that prescription drugs kill around 106,000 people in the US every year, which ranks prescription drugs as the fourth leading cause of death. Furthermore, each year sees 2,216,000 serious adverse drug reactions (defined as "those that required hospitalization, were permanently disabling, or resulted in death"). The authors of this 1998 study performed a meta-analysis on 39 previous studies covering 32 years. They factored out such things as medication errors, abuse of prescription drugs, and adverse reactions not considered serious. Plus, the study involved only people who had either been hospitalized due to drug reactions or who experienced reactions while in the hospital. People who died immediately (and, thus, never went to the hospital) and those whose deaths weren't realized to be due to prescription drugs were not included, so the true figure is probably higher. Four years later, another study in the JAMA warned:

Patient exposure to new drugs with unknown toxic effects may be extensive. Nearly 20 million patients in the United States took at least 1 of the 5 drugs withdrawn from the market between September 1997 and September 1998. Three of these 5 drugs were new, having been on the market for less than 2 years. Seven drugs approved since 1993 and subsequently withdrawn from the market have been reported as possibly contributing to 1002 deaths.

Examining warnings added to drug labels through the years, the study's authors found that of the new chemical entities approved from 1975 to 1999, 10 percent "acquired a new black box warning or were withdrawn from the market" by 2000. Using some kind of high-falutin' statistical process, they estimate that the "probability of a new drug acquiring black box warnings or being withdrawn from the market over 25 years was 20%." A statement released by one of the study's co-authors, Sidney Wolfe, MD, Director of Public Citizen's Health Studies Group, warned:

'In 1997, 39 new drugs were approved by the FDA. As of now [May 2002], five of them (Rezulin, Posicor, Duract, Raxar and Baycol) have been taken off the market and an additional two (Trovan, an antibiotic and Orgaran, an anticoagulant) have had new box warnings. Thus, seven drugs approved that year (18%

of the 39 drugs approved) have already been withdrawn or had a black box warning in just four years after approval. Based on our study, 20% of drugs will be withdrawn or have a black box warning within 25 years of coming on the market. The drugs approved in 1997 have already almost "achieved" this in only four years — with 21 years to go.' How does this happen? Before the FDA approves a new drug, it must undergo clinical trials. These trials aren't performed by the FDA, though — they're done by the drug companies themselves. These trials often use relatively few patients, and they usually select patients most likely to react well to the drug. On top of that, the trials are often for a short period of time (weeks), even though real-world users may be on a drug for months or years at a time. Dr. Wolfe points out that even when adverse effects show up during clinical trials, the drugs are sometimes released anyway, and they end up being taken off the market because of those same adverse effects. Post-marketing reporting of adverse effects isn't much better. The FDA runs a program to collect reports of problems with drugs, but compliance is voluntary. The generally accepted estimate in the medical community is that a scant 10 percent of individual instances of adverse effects are reported to the FDA, which would mean that the problem is ten times worse than we currently believe. Drugs aren't released when they've been proven safe; they're released when enough FDA bureaucrats — many of whom have worked for the pharmaceutical companies or will work for them in the future — can be convinced that it's kinda safe. Basically, the use of prescription drugs by the general public can be seen as widespread, long-term clinical trials to determine their true safety. We are all guinea pigs."

From 50 Things You're Not Supposed to Know by Russ Kick, published by The Disinformation Company Ltd. http://www.disinfo.com/

Note: Heroin – that most notorious of 'illegal', 'non-prescription' drugs, was originally developed by the pharmaceutical company BAYER for use as a legal prescription drug.

"The majority of the cancer patients in this country die because of chemotherapy, which does not cure breast, colon or lung cancer. This has been documented for over a decade and nevertheless doctors still utilize chemotherapy to fight these tumors." Allen Levin, MD, UCSF

"Several full-time scientists at the McGill Cancer Center sent to 118 doctors, all experts on lung cancer, a questionnaire to determine the level of trust they had in the therapies they were applying; they were asked to imagine that they themselves had contracted the disease and which of the six current experimental therapies they would choose. 79 doctors answered, 64 of them said that they would not consent to undergo any treatment containing cis-platinum – one of the common chemotherapy drugs they used – while 58 out of 79 believed that all the experimental therapies above were not accepted because of the ineffectiveness and the elevated level of toxicity of chemotherapy."

Philip Day, Cancer: why we're still dying to know the truth, Credence 2000

"If I were to contract cancer, I would never turn to a certain standard for the therapy of this disease. Cancer patients who stay away from these centers have some chance to make it."

Professor Gorge Mathe, Scientific Medicine Stymied, Medicines Nouvelles, Paris, 1989

"Dr. Hardin Jones, lecturer at the University of California, after having analyzed for many decades statistics on cancer survival, has come to this conclusion: '... when not treated, the patients do not get worse or they even get better'. The unsettling conclusions of Dr. Jones have never been refuted".

Walter Last, "The Ecologist", Vol. 28, no. 2, March-April 1998 ADVERSE DRUG REACTIONS: How Serious Is the Problem and How Often and Why Does It Occur?

"Although some adverse drug reactions are not very serious, others cause the death, hospitalization, or serious injury of more than 2 million people in the United states each year, including more than 100,000 fatalities. In fact, adverse drug reactions are one of the leading causes of death in the United States.' Most of the time, these dangerous events could and should have been avoided. Even the less drastic reactions, such as change in mood, loss of appetite, and nausea, may seriously diminish the quality of life. Despite the fact that more adverse reactions occur in patients 60 or older, the odds of suffering an adverse drug reaction really begin to increase even before age 50. Almost half (49.5%) of Food and Drug Administration (FDA) reports of deaths from adverse drug reactions and 61% of hospitalizations from adverse drug reactions were in people younger than 60.2 Many physical changes that affect the way the body can handle drugs actually begin in people in their thirties, but the increased prescribing of drugs does not begin for most people until they enter their fifties. By then, the amount of prescription drug use starts increasing significantly, and therefore the odds of having an adverse drug reaction also increase. The risk of an adverse drug reaction is about 33% higher in people aged 50 to 59 than it is in people aged 40."

Adverse Reactions to Drugs Cause Hospitalization of 1.5 Million Americans Each Year:

"An analysis of numerous studies in which the cause of hospitalization was determined found that approximately 1.5 million hospitalizations a year were caused by adverse drug reactions. This means that every day more than 9,000 patients have adverse drug reactions so serious that they need to be admitted to American hospitals. Although the rate of drug-induced hospitalization is higher in older adults (an average of about 10% of all hospitalizations for older adults are caused by adverse drug reactions) because they use more drugs, a significant proportion of hospitalizations for children is also caused by adverse drug reactions. In a review of more than 6,500 admissions of children to five different hospitals, 2.0% were prompted by adverse drug reactions."

Adverse Reactions Occur to 770,000 People a Year During Hospitalization

"In addition to the 1.5 million people a year who are admitted to the hospital because of adverse drug reactions, an additional three quarters of a million people a year develop an adverse reaction after they are hospitalized. According to national projection, based on a study involving adverse drug reactions developing in almost 800,000 patients a year, more than 2,000 patients a day, suffer an adverse event caused by drugs once they are admitted. Many of the reactions in the patients studied were serious, even life-threatening, and included cardiac arrhythmias, kidney failure, bleeding, and dangerously low blood pressure. People with these adverse reactions had an almost twofold higher risk of death compared to otherwise comparable hospitalized patients who did not have a drug reaction. Most importantly, according to the researchers, almost 50% of these adverse reactions were preventable. Among the kinds of preventable problems were adverse interactions between drugs that should not have been prescribed together (hundreds of these are listed in Chapter 3 of this book), known allergies to drugs that had not been asked about before the patients got a prescription, and excessively high doses of drugs prescribed without considering the patient's weight and kidney functions.

Thus, adding the number of people with adverse drug reactions so serious that they require hospitalization to those in which the adverse reaction was "caused" by the hospitalization, more than 2.2 million people a year, or 6,000 patients a day, suffer these adverse reactions. In both situations, many of these drug-induced problems should have been prevented."

Dr. Tim O'Shea, www.cancer-healing.com/pharma_pills.php

"...at least 250,000 people have attempted suicide worldwide because of Prozac alone and that at least 25,000 have succeeded."

Professor David Healy

5. From 'Doctor-Patient Communication: A Review'

Jennifer Fong Ha, MBBS (Hons) Dip Surg Anat and Nancy Longnecker, PhD, The Ochsner Journal, Ochsner Clinic Foundation, Spring 2010

"The patient will never care how much you know, until they know how much you care."

Terry Canale in his American Academy of Orthopaedic Surgeons Vice Presidential Address

Much patient dissatisfaction and many complaints are due to breakdown in the doctor-patient relationship. However, many doctors tend to overestimate their ability in communication.

Basic communication skills in isolation are insufficient to create and sustain a successful therapeutic doctor-patient relationship, which consists of shared perceptions and feelings regarding the nature of the problem, goals of treatment, and psychosocial support.

Studies on doctor-patient communication have demonstrated patient discontent even when many doctors considered the communication adequate or even excellent. Doctors tend to overestimate their abilities in communication. Tongue et al reported that 75% of the orthopedic surgeons surveyed believed that they communicated satisfactorily with their patients, but only 21% of the patients reported satisfactory communication with their doctors. Patient surveys have consistently shown that they want better communication with their doctors.

A more patient-centered encounter results in better patient as well as doctor satisfaction. Satisfied patients are less likely to lodge formal complaints or initiate malpractice complaints. Satisfied patients are advantageous for doctors in terms of greater job satisfaction, less work-related stress, and reduced burnout.

It has been observed that communication skills tend to decline as medical students progress through their medical education, and over time doctors in training tend to lose their focus on holistic patient care. Furthermore, the emotional and physical brutality of medical training, particularly during internship and residency, suppresses empathy, substitutes techniques and procedures for talk, and may even result in derision of patients.

Good communication skills practiced by doctors allowed patients to perceive themselves as a full participant during discussions relating to their health. This subjective experience that influences patient biology is the "biology of self-confidence" described by Sobel, which emphasized the critical role of patients' perception in their healing process.

There are reported observations of doctors avoiding discussion of the emotional and social impact of patients' problems because it distressed them when they could not handle these issues or they did not have the time to do so adequately. This situation negatively affected doctors emotionally and tended to increase patients' distress. This avoidance behavior may result in patients being unwilling to disclose problems, which could delay and adversely impact their recovery.

Physicians have been found to discourage patients from voicing their concerns and expectations as well as requests for more information. This negative influence of the doctors' behavior and the resultant nature of the doctor-patient communication deterred patients from asserting their need for information and explanations. Patients can feel disempowered and may be unable to achieve their health goals. Lack of sufficient explanation results in poor patient understanding, and a lack of consensus between doctor and patient may lead to therapeutic failure.

Today, patients have recognized that they are not passive recipients and are able to resist the power and expert authority that society grants doctors. They can implicitly and explicitly resist the monologue of information transfer from doctors by actively reconstructing expert information to assert their own perspectives, integrate with their knowledge of their own bodies and experiences, as well as the social realities of their lives. Being attentive to social relationships and contexts will ensure that this information is received, and most importantly, acted on.

...inequality, social relations, and structural constraints may be the most influential factors in health care.

Attentive listening skills, empathy, and use of open-ended questions are some examples of skillful communication.

Important factors include understanding patients' perspectives, sharing information, and patients' knowledge and expectations. Miscommunication has serious implications, as it may hinder patients' understanding, expectations of treatment, or involvement in treatment planning. In addition, miscommunication decreases patient satisfaction with medical care, level of hopefulness, and subsequent psychological adjustment.

...patients often regard their doctors as one of their most important sources of psychological support. Empathy is one of the most powerful ways of providing this support to reduce patients' feelings of isolation and validating their feelings or thoughts as normal and to be expected.

In addition to minimizing avoidance behavior, which prevents patients from expressing opinions, effective doctor-patient communication should involve productive conversation, which involves understanding of both parties' perspectives, by shifting from a perspective that is rigidly certain of one's belief to a more exploratory approach that strives to understand the situation from another perspective.

Good doctor-patient communication is a mechanism used to gain an understanding of patients' social context, expectations, and experience.

Doctor-patient communication is a major component of the process of health care. Doctors are in a unique position of respect and power. Hippocrates suggested that doctors may influence patients' health.

6. Extracts from
'The Way Toward Health' by Jane Roberts

If people become ill, it is quite fashionable to say that the immunity system has temporarily failed – yet the body itself knows that certain 'dis-eases' are healthy reactions. The body does not recognise <u>diseases as diseases</u> in usually understood terms. It regards all activity as experience, as a momentary condition of life, as a balancing situation.

It is ... fashionable to say that men and women have conscious minds, subconscious minds and unconscious minds – but there is no such thing as an unconscious mind. The body consciousness is <u>highly conscious</u>. You are simply not conscious of it.

You might say [instead] that varying portions of your own consciousness operate at different speeds. Translations between one portion of consciousness and another go on constantly, so that information is translated from one 'speed' to another.

....

Many psychiatrists and psychologists now realise that a disturbed client cannot be helped sufficiently unless the individual is considered along with his or her relationship to the family unit.

The same idea applies to physical illness as well. It is possible, however, to carry this idea even further, so that a person in poor health <u>should be</u> seen by the physician in relationship to the family and also in relationship to the environment. Old-time family doctors understood the patient's sensitivity to family members and to the environment, of course, and they often felt a lively sympathy and understanding that the practitioners of modern medicine often seem to have forgotten.

....

Modern medical science largely considers the human body to be a kind of mechanical model, a sort of vehicle like a car that needs to be checked by a garage every so often.

As an automobile is put together at an assembly line, so the body is seen as a very efficient machine put together in nature's 'factory'. If all the parts are in their proper place, and functioning smoothly, then the machine should give as excellent a service as any well-running automobile – or so it seems.

All of the automobile's parts, however, are alone responsible for its operations so long as it has a responsible driver. There are, however, hidden relationships that exist between various parts of the body – and the parts themselves are hardly mechanical. They change in every moment.

The heart is often described as a type of pump. With the latest developments in modern technology, there are all kinds of heart operations that can be performed, even the use of heart transplants. In many cases, even when hearts are repaired through medical technology, the same trouble reoccurs at a later date, or the patient recovers only to fall prey to a different, nearly fatal or fatal disease. This is not always the case by any means, but when such a person does recover fully, and maintains good health, it is because [their] beliefs, attitudes and feelings have changed for the better, and because the person 'has a heart' again; in other words because the patient himself has regained the will to live.

Many people who have heart trouble feel that they have 'lost the heart' for life. They may feel broken-hearted for many reasons. They may feel heartless, or imagine themselves to be so cold-hearted that they punish themselves literally by trying to lose their heart.

With many people having such difficulties, the addition of love in the environment may work far better than any heart operation. A new pet given to a bereaved individual has saved more people from needing heart operations than any physician. In other words, a 'love transplant' in the environment may work far better overall than a heart-transplant operation, or a bypass, or whatever; in such ways the heart is allowed to heal itself.

People have been taught to trust 275a picture of what is happening in their bodies, and cautioned not to trust their own feelings. Some public-service announcements stress the 'fact' that the individual can be gravely threatened by high blood pressure, for example, even though he or she feels in excellent health.

In many cases people exercise quite simply because they are afraid of what will happen if they do not. They may run to avoid heart disease, for example, whilst their own fear can <u>help</u> to promote the very eventuality they fear.

The body's health is an expression of inner well-being. Poor health is an expression also, and it may serve many purposes. It goes without saying that some people become ill rather than change their activities and their environments. They may also become ill, of course, to <u>force</u> themselves to make such changes.

I do not mean to imply that exercise is detrimental to good health. It is true, however, that the reason you exercise is more important than the exercises that you do perform. The reason can promote your good health or actually impede it.

....

The concept of survival of the fittest has had a considerable detrimental effect in many areas of human activity – particularly the realm of medical ideology and practice.

Politically as well as medically, such distortions have led to unfortunate conditions; the Aryan supremacy biological ideas fostered in the second world war, the concentration upon 'the perfect body', and other distortions. The idea of the ideal body has often been held up to the populace at large, and this often sets forth a stylised 'perfect' physique that actually could be matched by few individuals.

Any variations are frowned upon, and any birth defects considered in the most suspicious of lights. Some schools of thought then, have it that only the genetically superior should be allowed to reproduce, and there are scientists who believe that all defects can be eliminated through judicious genetic planning.

The handicapped are often given messages, even by the medical profession, that make them feel like misfits, unworthy to survive.

....

Your ideas about yourself are, again vital in the larger context of a healthy lifetime. The condition of your heart is affected, for example, by your own feelings about it. If you consider yourself to be cold-hearted or heartless, those feelings will have a significant effect upon that physical organ. If you feel broken-hearted then you will also have that feeling reflected in one way or another in the physical organ itself.

.... each individual also has many options open. Everyone who feels broken-hearted does not necessarily die of heart failure for example. The subject of health cannot be considered in an isolated fashion ... each person will try to fulfil their own unique abilities, and to 'fill out' the experience of life as fully as possible.

If an individual is hampered in that attempt strongly and persistently, then the dissatisfaction and frustration will be transformed into a lack of physical exuberance and vitality. There is always an unending reservoir of energy at the command of each person however, regardless of circumstances. ...

....

Thoughts and beliefs do indeed bring about physical alterations. They can even – and often do – change genetic message s.

There are diseases that people believe are inherited, carried from one generation to another by a faulty genetic communication. Obviously, many people with, for example, a genetic heritage of arthritis, do not come down with the disease themselves, while others indeed are so afflicted. The difference is one of belief.

The people who have accepted the suggestion uncritically that they will inherit such a malady do then seem to inherit it: they experience the symptoms. Actually the belief itself may have turned a healthy genetic message into an unhealthy one.

....

...pain and suffering are also obviously vital, living sensations – and therefore are a part of the body's repertoire of possible feelings and sensual experience. They are also a sign, therefore, of life's vitality, and are in themselves often responsible for a return to health when they act as learning communications.

Many diseases are often health-promoting processes. Chicken pox, measles and other like diseases in childhood in their own way 'naturally inoculate' the body, so that it is able to handle other elements that are a part of the body and the body's environment.

When civilised children are medically inoculated against such diseases ... to an important extent the natural protective processes are impeded. Such children may not come down with the disease against which they are medically protected, then – but they may indeed therefore become 'prey' to other diseases later in life that would not otherwise have occurred.

I am not advising people to refuse to have their children vaccinated, since you now have to take vaccination into consideration because of its prominence in society. It is very possible however, that science itself will in time discover the unfortunate side effects of many such procedures, and begin to reevaluate the entire subject.

....

... no person dies ahead of his or her time. The individual chooses the time of death. It is true however, that many cancers and conditions such as AIDS result because the immunity system has been so tampered with that the body has not been allowed to follow through with its own balancing act.

Again, however, no individual dies of cancer or AIDS, or any other condition, until they themselves have set the time.

...no consciousness considers death an end or a disaster, but views it instead as a means to the continuation of ... existence.

....

People with life-threatening diseases ... often feel that further growth, development, or expansion are highly difficult, if not impossible to achieve at a certain point in their lives. Often there are complicated family relationships that the person does not know how to handle ... In all cases, however, the need for value fulfilment, expression, and creativity are so important to life that when these are threatened, life itself is at least momentarily weakened. Innately, each person does realise that there is life after death, and in some instances such people realise that it is indeed time to move to another level of reality, to die and set out again with another brand new world.

Often, seriously ill people quite clearly recognise such feelings but they have been taught not to speak of them. The desire to die is considered cowardly, even evil, by some religions – and yet behind that desire lies all of the vitality of the will to life, which may already be seeking new avenues of expression and meaning.

There are those who come down with one serious disease – say heart trouble – who are cured through a heart transplant or other medical procedure, only to fall prey to another, seemingly unrelated disease, such as cancer. It would relieve the minds of family and friends, however if they understood that the individual involved did not 'fall prey' to the disease, and that he or she was not a victim in <u>usual</u> terms.

This does not mean that anyone consciously decides to get such-and-such a disease, but it does mean that some people instinctively realise that their own development <u>does</u> now demand another new framework of existence.

Much loneliness results when people who know they are going to die feel unable to communicate with loved ones for fear of hurting their feelings. Still other kinds of individuals will live long productive lives even while their physical mobility or health is most severely impaired. They will still feel that they had work to do, or that they were needed ...

....

Many cancer patients have martyr-like characteristics, often putting up with undesirable situations or conditions for years.

They feel powerless, unable to change, yet unwilling to stay in the same position. The most important point is to arouse such a person's belief in his or her strength and power. In many instances these people shrug their shoulders, saying "What will happen, will happen," but they do not physically struggle against their situation.

It is also vital that these patients are not overly medicated, for oftentimes the side effects of some cancer-eradicating drugs are dangerous in themselves. There has been some success with people who imagine that the cancer is instead some hated enemy or monster or foe, which is then banished with mental mock battles over a period of time. While the technique does have its advantages, it also pits one portion of the self against the other. It is much better to imagine say, the cancer cells being neutralised by some imaginary wand.

Doctors might suggest that a patient relax and then ask himself or herself what kind of inner fantasy would best serve the healing process. Instant images may come to mind at once, but if success is not achieved immediately, have the patient try again, for in almost all cases <u>some</u> inner picture will be perceived.

Behind the entire problem, however, is the fear of using one's full power or energy. Cancer patients most usually feel an inner impatience as they sense their own need for future expansion and development, only to feel it thwarted.

Again, we cannot generalise overmuch, but many persons know quite well that they are not sure whether they want to live or die. The overabundance of cancer cells represents nevertheless the need for expression and expansion – the only arena left open – or so it would seem.

Such a person must also contend with society's unfortunate ideas about the disease in general, so that many cancer patients end up isolated or alone. As in almost all cases of disease however, if it were possible to have a kind of 'thought transplant' operation, the disease would quickly vanish.

Consciously you might want to express certain abilities, whilst unconsciously you are afraid of doing so.

....

For all of life's seeming misfortunes, development, fulfilment and accomplishment far outweigh death, diseases and disasters. Starting over can be done – by anyone in any situation, and it will bring about some beneficial effects regardless of previous conditions.

Behind all maladies, in the most basic manner lies the need for expression, and when people feel that their areas of growth are being curtailed, then they instigate actions meant to clear the road, so to speak.

Before health problems show up there is almost always a loss of self-respect or expression.

In the matter of the disease called AIDS, for example, you have groups of homosexuals, many 'coming out of the closet' for the first time, taking part in organisations that promote their cause, and suddenly faced by the suspicions and distrust of many other portions of the population.

The struggle to express themselves, and their own unique abilities and characteristics, drives them on, and yet is all too frequently thwarted by the ignorance and misunderstanding that surrounds them. You end up with something like a psychological contagion. The people involved begin to feel even more depressed as they struggle to combat the prejudice against them. Many of them almost hate themselves. For all their seeming bravado, they fear that they are indeed unnatural members of the species.

These beliefs break down the immunity system and bring about the symptoms so connected with the disease. AIDS is a social phenomenon to that extent, expressing the deep dissatisfactions, doubts and angers of a prejudiced-against segment of society.

Whatever physical changes occur, happen because the will to live is weakened. AIDS is a kind of biological protest, as if the homosexuals are saying: "You may as well kill us. We might be better off than the way you treat us now" ...

The attitude of doctors and nurses towards the handling of such patients shows only too clearly not only their fear of the disease itself, but their fear of homosexuality, which has been considered evil and forbidden by many religions.

Yet AIDS can be acquired by those who are not homosexuals, but who have similar problems. It is a great error to segregate some individuals, like a modern colony of lepers.

Many other conditions that seem to be spread by viruses or contagions are also related to the problems of society in the same manner, and when these conditions are righted the diseases themselves largely vanish. It should be remembered that it is the beliefs and feelings of the patients that largely determine the effectiveness of any medical procedures, techniques or medications.

Unfortunately, the entire picture surrounding health and disease is a largely negative one, in which even preventative medicine can have severe drawbacks, since it often recommends drugs or techniques to attack a problem not only before the problem emerges, but simply in case it emerges.

Many of the public-health announcements routinely publicise the specific symptoms of various diseases, almost as if laying out maps of diseases for medical consumers to follow.

The body's own healing processes are forever active however – which is why I so strongly advise them being relied upon along with whatever medical help seems appropriate. But the individual, even as a patient, must always have a choice, and the right to refuse any treatment being offered.

....

You cannot divorce philosophy from life, for your thoughts and opinions give your life its meaning and impetus. There are some people who believe that life is meaningless, that it has no purpose, and that its multitudinous parts fell together through the workings of chance alone. Obviously I am speaking of scientific dogma, but such dogma is far more religious than scientific, for it also expects to be believed without proof, on faith alone.

All of life is seen as heading for extinction in any case. The entire concept of a soul, life after death, or even life from one generation to the next, becomes doubtful, to say the least. In such a philosophical world it would seem that man has no power at all.

... those concepts can have a hand in the development of would-be suicides, particularly of a young age, for they seem to effectively block a future.

....

For centuries it was taken for granted that God was on the side of the strongest, richest nation. Surely, it seemed, if a country was poor or downtrodden, it was because God made it so.

Such ideas literally held people in chains, fostering slavery and other inhumane practices. The same unfortunately applies to Eastern concepts of nirvana and to the Christian idea of heaven.

There are many differences between the ideas of nirvana and heaven, but each has been used, not only to justify suffering, but also to teach people to seek pain.

Quite ordinary people often believe, then, that suffering itself is a way towards personal development and spiritual knowledge. In matters of health, such beliefs can have most unfortunate results. They are often responsible for needless sacrifices of physical organs in imprudent operations.

Some individuals become anxious and worried if they think they are too happy – for them it means they are not paying sufficiently for their sins. They may be threatened by some undeniable danger, until finally, in one way or another they seek out their own punishment once again – wondering all the time why they are so frequently besieged by poor health or disease.

This kind of syndrome can affect individuals, families, and to some extent entire nations. They mitigate directly against man's health, survival and exuberance.

Constant fears about … catastrophes can also fall under this classification.

This is true of individuals, but it also applies to many so-called survival groups, who congregate in one or another portion of the country.

Most such people expect a period of chaotic time, in which all laws are broken down. Another version stresses the economic area, foreseeing the collapse of the economy, anarchy, and other conditions that pit one individual against another. Some use religious dogma and others rely upon scientific dogma to prove their cases ...

Good mental or physical health can hardly flourish in such conditions.

Such ideas affect every level of life, from the most microscopic onward. It is not that plants understand your ideas in usual terms, but that they do indeed pick up your intent, and in the area of world survival, they have a stake.

I do not want to romanticise nonhuman life either, or to overestimate its resources, but nature also has its own ways – and in those ways it constantly works towards the survival of life in general. Nature <u>may not bail you out</u>, but it will always be there, adding its own vitality and strength to the overall good and health of the planet.

Communication flashes between viruses and microbes, and they can change in the wink of an eye. Once again then, ideas of the most optimistic nature are the biologically pertinent ones.

....

This is a good place to bring up some extreme food practices, such as over-fasting and an obsession with so-called natural foods. I am not talking about a natural and healthy interest in the purity of foodstuffs, but of a worrisome overconcern.

Behind many such attitudes is the idea that the body itself is unworthy, and that starving it somehow cuts down on the appetites of the flesh. You usually end up with a flurry of different types of diets.

Some concentrate almost exclusively on protein, some on carbohydrates – particularly rice – but in any case the large natural range of foods and nutrients are cut out.

This keeps the body in a state of constant turmoil. Some people are so convinced, in fact, that eating is wrong that they diet until they become ravenously hungry, then overeat and force themselves to vomit up the residue.

Other people, in a well-meaning attempt to watch their weight, skip their breakfasts entirely – a very poor procedure.

It is far better to eat moderate amounts of food in all of the food ranges, and to consume smaller portions more often ... <u>four light meals a day</u> will overall serve you very well.

These food ideas are important, since they are often passed on from parents to children, and parents often use food as a way of rewarding a child's good behaviour, thus starting the youngster out towards the condition of overweight.

....

If you do have health problems, it is much better to look for their reason in your immediate experience ...

... try to understand that the particular dilemma of illness is not an event forced upon you by some other agency. Rather realise that to some extent or another your dilemma or your illness <u>has been chosen by you</u> ...

If you realise that your beliefs form your experience, then you do have a very good chance of changing your beliefs, and hence your experience.

You can discover what your own reasons are for choosing the dilemma or illness by being very honest with yourself. There is no need to feel guilty since you <u>meant very well</u> as you made each choice – only the choices were built upon beliefs that were beliefs and <u>not facts</u>.

If you are in serious difficulties of any kind, it may at first seem inconceivable, unbelievable or even scandalous to imagine that your problems are caused by your beliefs. In fact, the opposite may appear to be true. You might have lost a series of jobs, and it may seem quite clear to you that you are not to blame in any of these circumstances.

You may be in the middle of one or several unsatisfactory relationships, none of which seem to be caused by you, while instead you believe you are an unwilling victim or participant. You may have a dangerous drug or alcohol problem, or you may be married to someone who does.

In most cases, even the most severe illnesses or complicated living conditions are caused by an attempt to grow, develop or expand in the face of difficulties that appear to be insurmountable to one degree or another.

An individual will appear to be striving for some goal that appears blocked, and hence he or she uses all available energy and strength to circumnavigate the blockage.

[In fact] the blockage is usually a belief which needs to be understood or removed rather than bypassed.

....

You are not healthy ... no matter how robust your physical condition, if your relationships are unhealthy, unsatisfying, frustrating or hard to achieve. Whatever your situation is, it is a good idea to ask yourself <u>what you would do</u> if you were free of it. An alcoholic's wife might wish with all her heart that her husband would stop drinking – but if she suddenly asked herself what she would do, she might – surprisingly enough –

feel a tinge of panic. On examination of her own thoughts and feelings, she might well discover that she was so frightened of not achieving her own goals that she actually encouraged her husband's alcoholism, so that she would not have to face her own 'failure'. Obviously this hypothetical situation is a quick example of what I mean, with no mention of the innumerable other beliefs and half-beliefs that would encircle the man's and the woman's relationship.

Each person is so unique that it is obviously impossible for me to discuss all of the innumerable strands of belief that form human experience .... you may discover not just one you, but several you's, so to speak, each pursuing certain purposes, and you may find out furthermore that some purposes cancel others out, whilst some are diametrically opposed to one another. Such cross-purposes, of course can lead to mental, spiritual, emotional and physical difficulties.

Large numbers of people do indeed live unsatisfactory lives, with many individuals seeking goals that are nearly unattainable because of the conglomeration of contradictory beliefs that vie for their attention. They are at cross-purposes with themselves.

Addendum: from 'The Individual and the Nature of Mass Events' – a Seth Book by Jane Roberts :

Many therefore "fall prey" to epidemics of one kind or another because they want to, though they might deny this quite vigorously.

I am speaking particularly of epidemics that are less than deadly, though danger is involved. In your times, hospitals, you must realize, are important parts of the community. They provide a social as well as a medical service. Many people are simply lonely, or overworked. Some are rebelling against commonly held ideas of competition. Flu epidemics become social excuses for much needed rest, therefore, and serve as face-saving devices so that the individual can hide from *themselves* their inner difficulties. In a way, such epidemics provide their own kind of fellowship – giving common meeting grounds for those of disparate circumstances. The [epidemics] serve as accepted states of illness, in which people are given an excuse for the rest or quiet self-examination they desperately need but do not feel entitled to otherwise.

I do not mean to assign any hint of accusation against those so involved, but mainly to state some of the reasons for such behavior. If you do not trust your nature, then any illness or disposition will be interpreted as an onslaught against health. Your body faithfully reflects your inner psychological reality. The nature of your emotions means that in the course of a lifetime you will experience the full range of feelings. Your subjective state has variety. Sometimes sad or depressing thoughts provide a refreshing change of pace, leading you to periods of quiet reflection, and to a quieting of the body so that it rests.

Fears, sometimes even seemingly irrational ones, can serve to rouse the body if you have been too lethargic, or have been in a rut psychologically or physically. If you trusted your nature you would be able to trust such feelings, and following their own rhythms and routes they would change into others. Ideally even illnesses are a part of the body's health, representing needed adjustments, and also following the needs of the subjective person at any given time.

7. Extracts from 'Medical Nemesis – The Expropriation of Health' by Ivan Illich

The medical establishment has become a major threat to health. The disabling impact of professional control over medicine has reached the proportions of an epidemic. *Iatrogenesis,* the name for this new epidemic, comes from *iatros,* the Greek word for 'physician', and *genesis,* meaning 'origin'.

A professional and physician-based health-care system that has grown beyond critical bounds is sickening for three reasons: it must produce clinical damage that outweighs its potential benefits; it cannot but enhance even as it obscures the political conditions that render society unhealthy; and it tends to expropriate the power of the individual to heal himself and shape his or her environment.

More and more people subconsciously know that they are sick and tired of their jobs and of their leisure passivities, but they want to hear the lie that physical illness relieves them of social and political responsibilities. They want their doctor to act as lawyer and priest. As a lawyer, the doctor exempts the patient from his normal duties and enables him to cash in on the insurance fund he was forced to build. As a priest, he becomes the patient's accomplice in creating the myth that he is an innocent victim of biological mechanisms rather than a lazy, greedy or envious deserter of a social struggle for control over the tools of production. Social life becomes a giving and receiving of therapy: medical, psychiatric, pedagogic or geriatric.

People who are angered, sickened and impaired by their industrial labour and leisure can escape only into a life under medical supervision and are thereby seduced or disqualified from political struggle for a healthier world.

Medicine has the authority to label one man's complaint a legitimate illness, to declare a second man sick though he does not himself complain, and to refuse a third social recognition of his pain, his disability and even his death. It is medicine which stamps some pain as 'merely subjective', some impairment as malingering, and some deaths – though not others – as suicide. The judge determines what is legal and who is guilty. The priest declares what is holy and who has broken a taboo. The physician decides what is a symptom and who is sick.

For rich and poor...life is reduced to a 'span', to a statistical phenomenon which, for better or worse, must be institutionally planned and shaped. This life-span is brought into existence with the pre-natal check-up...and it will end with a mark on a chart...

To be in good health means not only to be successful in coping with reality but also to enjoy the success; it means to be able to feel alive in pleasure and in pain; it means to cherish but also to risk survival. Health and suffering, as experienced sensations are phenomena that distinguish men from beasts. Only storybook lions are said to *suffer* and only pets to merit compassion when they are in ill-health.

Medicalisation constitutes a prolific bureaucratic programme based on the denial of each man's need to deal with pain, sickness and death. The modern medical enterprise represents an endeavour to do for people what their genetic and cultural heritage formerly equipped them to do for themselves. Medical civilization is planned and organized to kill pain, to eliminate sickness, and to abolish the need for an art of suffering and of dying.

Culture makes pain tolerable by interpreting its necessity; only pain perceived as curable is intolerable.

A myriad virtues express the different aspects of fortitude that traditionally enabled people to recognize painful sensations as a challenge and to shape their own experience accordingly. Patience, forbearance, courage, resignation, self-control, perseverance, and meekness each express a different colouring of the responses with which pain sensations were accepted, transformed into the experience of suffering and endured. Duty, love, fascination, routines, prayer, and compassion were some of the means that enabled pain to be borne with dignity.

The pupils of Hippocrates distinguished many kinds of disharmony, each of which caused its own type of pain...Pain might disappear in the process of healing, but this was certainly not the primary object of the...treatment. The Greeks did not even think about enjoying happiness without taking pain in their stride. Pain was the soul's experience of evolution...

The body had not yet been divorced from the soul, nor had sickness been divorced from pain. All words that indicated bodily pain were equally applicable to the suffering of the soul.

[The] raised threshold of physiologically mediated experience, which is characteristic of a medicalised society, makes it extremely difficult today to recognize in the capacity for suffering a possible symptom of health. The reminder that suffering is a responsible activity is almost unbearable to consumers, for whom pleasure and dependence on industrial outputs coincide.

During the 17th and 18th centuries, doctors who applied measurements to sick people were liable to be considered quacks by their colleagues. During the French Revolution, English doctors still looked askance at clinical thermometry, Together with the routine taking of the pulse, it became accepted clinical practice only around 1845, nearly thirty years after the stethoscope was first used by Laenne.

An advanced industrial society is sick-making because it disables people from coping with their environment and, when they break down, it substitutes a 'clinical' prosthesis for the broken *relationships.*

People would rebel against such an environment if medicine did not explain their biological disorientation as a defect in their health, rather than as a defect in the way of life which is imposed on them or which they impose on themselves.

The medical diagnosis of substantive disease entities that supposedly take shape in the individual's body is a surreptitious and amoral way of blaming the victim. The physician, himself a member of the dominating class, judges that the individual does not fit into an environment that has been engineered and is administered by other professionals, instead of accusing his colleagues of creating environments into which the human organism cannot fit.

Before sickness came to be perceived primarily as an organic or behavioural abnormality, he who got sick could still find in the eyes of the doctor a reflection of his own anguish and some recognition of the uniqueness of his suffering. Now, what he meets is the gaze of a biological accountant engaged in input/output calculations. His sickness is taken from him and turned into the raw material for an institutional enterprise. His condition is interpreted according to a set of abstract rules in a language he cannot understand. He is taught only about alien entities that the doctor combats, but only just as much as the doctor considers necessary to gain the patient's cooperation. Language is taken over by the doctors: the sick person is deprived of meaningful words for his anguish, which is thus further increased by linguistic mystification.

...while the industrial worker refers to his ache as a drab 'it' that hurts, his predecessors had many colourful and expressive names for the demons that bit or stung them.

Through the medicalisation of death, health care has become a monolithic world religion...

Like time-consuming acceleration, stupefying education, self-destructive military defence, disorienting information, or unsettling housing projects, pathogenic medicine is the result of industrial overproduction that paralyses autonomous action.

The patient is reduced to an object – his body – being repaired; he is no longer a subject being helped to heal. If he is allowed to participate in the repair process, he acts as the lowest apprentice in a hierarchy of repairmen. Often he is not even trusted to take a pill without the supervision of a nurse.

When people become aware of their dependence on the medical industry, they tend to be trapped in the belief that they are already hopelessly hooked. They fear a life of disease without a doctor much as they would feel immobilized without a car or bus.

Increasing and irreparable damage accompanies present industrial expansion in all sectors. In medicine this damage appears as iatrogenesis. Iatrogenesis is clinical when pain, sickness and death result from medical care; it is social when health policies reinforce an industrial organization that generates ill-health; it is cultural and symbolic when medically sponsored behaviour and delusions restrict the vital autonomy of people by undermining their competence in growing up, caring for each other, and aging, or when medical intervention cripples personal responses to pain, disability, impairment, anguish and death.

Man's consciously lived fragility, individuality, and relatedness make the experience of pain, of sickness, and of death an integral part of his life. The ability to cope with this trio autonomously is fundamental to his health. As he becomes dependent on the management of his intimacy, he renounces his autonomy and his health *must* decline. The true miracle of modern medicine is diabolical. It consists in making not only individuals but whole populations survive on inhumanly low levels of personal health. Medical nemesis is the negative feedback of a social organization that sets out to improve and equalize the opportunity for each man to cope in autonomy and ended by destroying it.

Further Reading and Web Resources

Avery, Samuel *The Dimensional Structure of Consciousness*

Avery, Samuel *Transcendence of the Western Mind*

Balint, Michael *The Doctor, His Patient and the Illness*

Boadella, David *Lifestreams*

Broom, Brian *Meaning-full Disease – How personal experience and meanings cause and maintain physical illness*

Broom, Brian *Somatic Illness and the Patient's Other Story*

Broom, Brian *Transforming Clinical Practice Using the MindBody Approach: A Radical Integration*

Carel, Havi *Illness*

Chiozza, Luis A. *Hidden Affects in Somatic Disorders*

Chiozza, Luis A. *Why Do We Fall Ill?*

Foucault, Michel *The Birth of the Clinic*

Goldstein, Kurt *The Organism*

Groddeck, G. *The Meaning of Illness.*

Heidegger, Martin *Zollikon Seminars*

Illich, Ivan *Limits to Medicine: Medical Nemesis – The Expropriation of Health*

Kay, Lily *Who Wrote the Book of Life?*

Kleinman, Arthur *The Illness Narratives*

Lakoff and Johnson, *Metaphors We Live By*

Lanctot, Guylaine *The Medical Mafia*

Leader, Darian and Cornfield, David *Why do People Get Ill?*

Lewontin, R. C. *Biology as Ideology*

Mindell, Arnold *Working with the Dreaming Body*

Roberts, Jane *The Way Toward Health - a Seth book*

Roberts, Janine *Fear of the Invisible*

Sveneaus, Sven *The Hermeneutics of Medicine and the Phenomenology of Health*

Tauber, Alfred I. *The Immune Self*

Welch, Dr. H. Gilbert *Overdiagnosed: Making People Sick in the Pursuit of Health*

Zigmond, David *If You Want Good Personal Healthcare See a Vet*

Web Resources

PeterWilberg www.peterwilberg.org

Life Medicine and Life Doctoring www.lifedoctoring.org.uk

Existential Medicine www.existentialmedicine.org

Martin Heidegger www.heidegger.org.uk

The New Therapy www.thenewtherapy.org.uk

The New Psychiatry www.thenewpsychiatry.org

The Awareness Principle www.theawarenessprinciple.com

Head, Heart and Hara http://headheartandhara.blogspot.com

Centre for Medical Humanities https://www.dur.ac.uk/cmh/

International Society of Logotherapy and Existential Analysis http://www.existential-analysis.org/

Darian Leader http://whydopeoplegetill.blogspot.co.uk

Iraq Society for Phenomenological Medicine https://www.facebook.com/Phenomedicine

International Federation of Daseinsanalysis http://www.daseinsanalyse.com/ifda/federation.html

Viktor von Weizsaecker Gesellschaft http://viktor-von-weizsaecker-gesellschaft.de/

The Balint Society http://balint.co.uk/

Dr David Zigmond www.davidzigmond.org.uk

http://www.april.org.uk– on adverse drug reactions

www.beyondmeds.com

Other Books and Articles by Peter Wilberg

from PSYCHOSOMATICS to SOMA-SEMIOTICS - Felt Sense and the Sensed Body in Medicine and Psychotherapy New Yoga Publications 2010

Heidegger, Medicine and 'Scientific Method'
New Gnosis Publications 2005

Meditation and Mental Health – an introduction to Awareness Based Cognitive Therapy
New Yoga Publications 2010

The Therapist as Listener – Heidegger and the Missing Dimension of Counselling and Psychotherapy Training
New Gnosis Publications 2005

The Awareness Principle – a Radical New Philosophy of Life, Science and Religion New Yoga Publications 2008

*The QUALIA Revolution – from Quantum Physics to Qualia Scien*ce Second Edition, New Gnosis Publications 2008

Tantra Reborn – The Sensuality and Sexuality of our Immortal Soul Body New Yoga Publications 2009

The New Yoga of Awareness – Tantric Wisdom for Today's World New Yoga Publications 2209

The Science Delusion – Why God is Real and Science is Religious Myth New Yoga Publications 2008

Event Horizon – Terror, Tantra and the Ultimate Metaphysics of Awareness New Yoga Publications 2008

Heidegger, Phenomenology and Indian Thought
NewYoga Publications 2008

Deep Socialism – A New Manifesto of Marxist Ethics and Economics New Gnosis Publications 2003

From New Age to New Gnosis – Towards a New Gnostic Spirituality New Gnosis Publications 2003

Head, Heart and Hara – the Soul Centres of West and East New Gnosis Publications, 2003

Articles:

The Language of Listening
Journal of the Society for Existential Analysis 3

Introduction to Maieutic Listening
Journal of the Society for Existential Analysis 8.1

Listening as Bodywork
Energy and Character; Journal of Biosynthesis 30/2

From Existential Psychotherapy to Existential Medicine Journal of the Society for Existential Analysis 22.2 July 2011

Index

www.ingramcontent.com/pod-product-compliance
Lightning Source LLC
Chambersburg PA
CBHW051439170526
45166CB00001B/50